Anatomy Studymate

Maps & Mnemonics

First edition

2015

Cover & internal design: Mina Azer

First edition: 2015

First Printing: March 2015

Printed by CreateSpace, An Amazon.com Company

ISBN-13: 978-1508887577

ISBN-10: 1508887578

FOCUS for capacity building solutions

www.focus4courses.blogspot.com

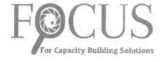

To my mother, wife and daughter.

My love, motive and hope.

M. A.

Author's Biography

Mina Azer got his MSc in surgery in 2013. He has a great passion for science yielded in his current research and publications. Between 2004 and 2014 he shared in more than 70 different training delivered to more than 2000 trainees about various topics such as: reproductive health, surgical skills, and medical research. He is currently working as a surgery specialist at the Egyptian Liver Research Institute and Hospital.

Contents

Preface

The idea of this book have been in my mind for at least 15 years. That is not a good thing to admit that I have been thinking a project over for one and a half decades. But the truth is that I never felt mature enough – knowledge wise- to start writing my own book. Then at last I had this thought few months ago: "if I am going to wait for my knowledge to complete, I will be kidding myself as there is no such thing." Here I decided to start writing what is the best to my knowledge.

This book is simply my study notes during my undergraduate study, then the exams for the master's degree in surgery, and finally the step A exam of the membership of the royal college of surgeons (MRCS). And don't worry, I passed them all, so you can depend on this book for a valid reason.

Anatomy Studymate is not meant to replace anatomy text books. Unless coffee mate was meant to replace coffee. Think of it like a side dish, that can't feed you alone. Yet, it adds a flavor to your meal.

Ok!! Enough coffee and dinner talk. Bottom line, this book can really help you in many ways. When you study a topic for the first time, it can offer you a simpler – or sometimes deeper insights. Writing the mnemonics in your main source next to each topic is a good idea. Also during revision, I think that condensing the important topics of anatomy in 150 low-text and details-free pages can be helpful. At last during your postgraduate study, this book can be particularly helpful to remember the highlights and the hot topics, which are always the core of exams like masters, PhD and even MRCS.

The User's Guide!!

This book has 5 chapters covering the main regions of the body: upper limb, lower limb, thorax, abdomen & pelvis and head & neck.

Each chapter is further divided to many sections marked by one of the following icons.

 The key is for a mnemonic.

 The globe is for a diagram.

 The table is for a table.

 The book is for a summary verse.

The topics were written in order as mentioned in the heading of each chapter. Notice that not all topics are covered, only those who are either extremely important or can be explained via a mnemonic, tables, diagram or a short paragraph.

Chapter 1: Upper Limb

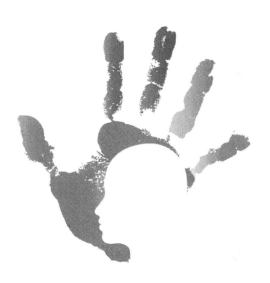

Contents

- Pectoral region and Axilla
- Arm
- Forearm
- Hand

Pectoral region & Axilla

1 Breast – Site

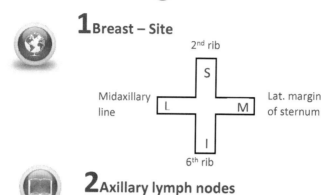

2 Axillary lymph nodes

Afferent: cubital nodes; lymphatic vessels from the upper limb, thoracic wall and subscapular region.

Efferent: efferent vessels form the subclavian trunk, some drainage to inferior deep cervical nodes.

Regions drained: upper limb, most of the mammary gland, some of the anterolateral chest wall, posterior thoracic wall and scapular region.

Formation: axillary nodes number from 20 to 30 and are organized in five groups based on their position within the axilla: 1) pectoral nodes, along the lateral border of the pectoralis major m.; 2) lateral nodes, located along the distal axillary v.; 3) central nodes, centrally located along axillary v.; 4) subscapular nodes, located along the subscapular v. and its tributaries; 5) apical nodes, located at the apex of axilla.

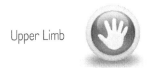

3 Breast – Lymphatic drainage

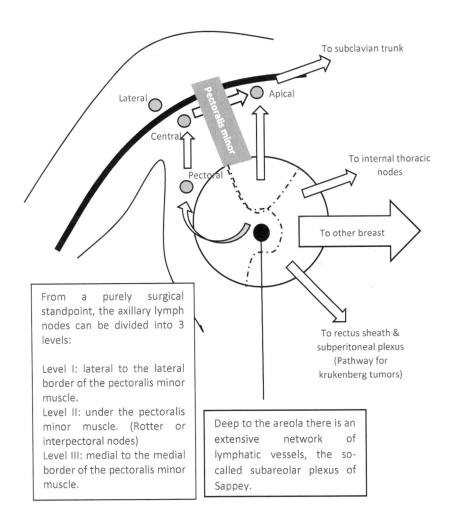

To subclavian trunk

Lateral

Pectoralis minor

Apical

Central

Pectoral

To internal thoracic nodes

To other breast

From a purely surgical standpoint, the axillary lymph nodes can be divided into 3 levels:

Level I: lateral to the lateral border of the pectoralis minor muscle.
Level II: under the pectoralis minor muscle. (Rotter or interpectoral nodes)
Level III: medial to the medial border of the pectoralis minor muscle.

To rectus sheath & subperitoneal plexus (Pathway for krukenberg tumors)

Deep to the areola there is an extensive network of lymphatic vessels, the so-called subareolar plexus of Sappey.

4Pectoral girdle muscles

	Muscle	Origin	Insertion	Action	Nerve	Notes
Pectoral Girdle Stabilizing muscles	pectoralis minor	ribs 3-5	coracoid process of the scapula	draws the scapula forward, medially, and downward	medial pectoral nerve (C8, T1)	branches of medial pectoral nerve usually pierce pectoralis minor to reach the pectoralis major muscle
	rhomboideus major	spines of vertebrae T2-T5	medial border of the scapula inferior to the spine of the scapula	retracts, elevates and rotates the scapula inferiorly	dorsal scapular nerve (C5)	named for its shape (rhomboid)
	rhomboideus minor	inferior end of the ligamentum nuchae, spines of vertebrae C7 and T1	medial border of the scapula at the root of the spine of the scapula			
	serratus anterior	ribs 1-8 or 9	medial border of the scapula on its costal (deep) surface	it draws the scapula forward; the inferior fibers rotate the scapula superiorly	long thoracic nerve (from ventral rami C5-C7)	a lesion of long thoracic nerve will cause winging of the scapula (i.e., like an angel's wing)
	trapezius	medial third of superior nuchal line, external occipital protuberance, ligamentum nuchae, spinous processes of vertebrae C7-T12	lateral third of the clavicle, medial side of the acromion and the upper crest of the scapular spine, tubercle of the scapular spine	elevates and depresses the scapula (depending on which part of the muscle contracts); rotates the scapula superiorly; retracts scapula	motor: spinal accessory (XI), proprioception: C3-C4	named for its shape; trapezius is an example of a muscle that migrates during development from its level of origin (cervical) to its final position, pulling its nerve and artery along behind

subclavius	first rib and its cartilage	inferior surface of the clavicle	draws the clavicle (and hence the shoulder) down and forward	nerve to subclavius (C5)	it serves an important protective function - it cushions the subclavian vessels from bone fragments in clavicular fractures

5 Pectoral nerves: Path of lateral vs. medial

"Lateral **L**ess, **M**edial **M**ore":
Lateral pectoral nerve only goes through Pectoralis major, but Medial pectoral nerve goes though both Pectoralis major and minor.

6 Serratus anterior: innervation and action

"**C5-6-7**
raise your **wings** up to **heaven**":
C**567** injury causes inability to **raise** arm past 90 degrees up to **heaven**, and results in a **winging** of the scapula.
Long thoracic nerve roots (567) innervate Serratus anterior.

7 Brachial plexus: numbers of each section

It is the same backwards and forwards:
5-3-2-3-5:
5 Roots
3 Trunks
2 Divisions
3 Cords
5 Terminal Nerves

8 Brachial plexus

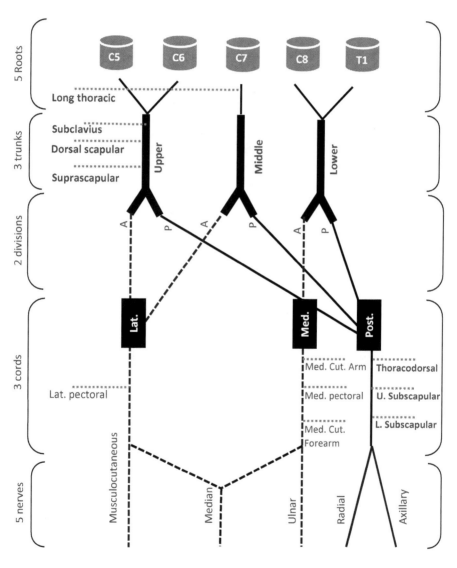

9 Brachial plexus: sections

"Nerves Climb Down Trees reaching **Roots"** - *backwards*

Terminal **Nerves**
Cords
Divisions
Trunks
Roots

10 Brachial plexus: branches of posterior cord

STAR:
Subscapular [upper and lower]
Thoracodorsal
Axillary
Radial

11 Shoulder joint

Synovial, ball & socket joint, connects humerus & scapula; glenoid labrum deepens the socket, glenohumeral ligaments located anteriorly; tendon of long head of biceps passes through shoulder joint, strengthened by the rotator cuff muscles.

Glenohumeral ligament

Inferior: capsular ligament connects humerus to scapula; represents an anteroinferior thickening of the shoulder joint capsule; weak support for joint.

Middle: capsular ligament connects humerus to scapula; represents an anterointermediate thickening of the shoulder joint capsule; weak support for joint.

Superior: capsular ligament connects humerus to scapula; represents an anterosuperior thickening of the shoulder joint capsule; weak support for joint.

 12Axillary artery

Divided into 3 parts by the pectoralis minor

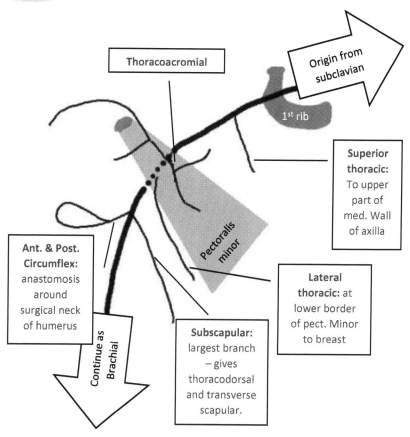

13 Axillary artery – branches

"Screw The Lawyer Save A Patient":

Superior thoracic
Thoracoacromial
Lateral thoracic
Subscapular
Anterior circumflex humeral
Posterior circumflex humeral

Alternatively: "Some Times Life Seems A Pain".

14 Thoracoacromial artery branches

ABCD:
Acromial
Breast (pectoral)
Clavicular
Deltoid

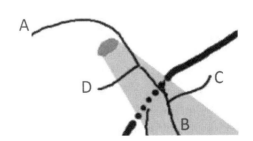

15 Transverse Scapular Ligament

Army over (bridge), Navy under (bridge)
Artery goes over (suprascapular artery) and **Nerve** goes under the ligament (suprascapular nerve).

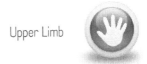

Arm

16 Muscles moving the arm

Muscles moving the arm	**pectoralis major**	medial 1/2 of the clavicle, manubrium & body of sternum, costal cartilages of ribs 2-6, sometimes from the rectus sheath of the upper abdominal wall	crest of the greater tubercle of the humerus	flexes and adducts the arm, medially rotates the arm	medial and lateral pectoral n (C5-T1)	deep fascia on its anterior surface should not be fused to the fascia of the mammary gland - if it is, this is an important clinical sign indicating breast disease
	latissimus dorsi	vertebral spines from T7 to the sacrum, posterior third of the iliac crest, lower 3 or 4 ribs, sometimes from the inferior angle of the scapula	floor of the intertubercular groove	extends the arm and rotates the arm medially	thoracodorsal nerve (C7,8)	the inserting tendon twists so that fibers originating highest insert lowest
	deltoid	lateral one-third of the clavicle, acromion, the lower lip of the crest of the spine of the scapula	deltoid tuberosity of the humerus	abducts arm; anterior fibers flex & medially rotate the arm; posterior fibers extend & laterally rotate the arm	axillary nerve (C5,6)	the deltoid muscle is the principle abductor of the arm but due to poor mechanical advantage it cannot initiate this action; it is assisted by the supraspinatus m.
	subscapularis	medial two-thirds of the costal surface of the scapula (subscapular fossa)	lesser tubercle of the humerus	medially rotates the arm; assists extension of the arm	upper and lower subscapular	subscapularis, supraspinatus, infraspinatus, and teres minor are the rotator cuff muscles

19

	Origin	Insertion	Action	Nerve	Notes
supraspinatus	supraspinatus fossa	greater tubercle of the humerus (highest facet)	abducts the arm (initiates abduction)	suprascapular nerve (C5,6)	supraspinatus initiates abduction of the arm, then the deltoid muscle completes the action; a member of the rotator cuff group
infraspinatus	infraspinatus fossa	greater tubercle of the humerus (middle facet)	laterally rotates the arm	suprascapular nerve	infraspinatus, supraspinatus, teres minor and subscapularis are the rotator cuff muscles
teres major	dorsal surface of the inferior angle of the scapula	crest of the lesser tubercle of the humerus	adducts the arm, medially rotates the arm, assists in arm extension	lower subscapular nerve (C5,6)	teres major inserts beside the tendon of latissimus dorsi, and assists latissimus in its actions
teres minor	upper 2/3 of the lateral border of the scapula	greater tubercle of the humerus (lowest facet)	laterally rotates the arm	axillary nerve (C5,6)	fixes the head of the humerus in the glenoid fossa during abduction & flexion of the arm; a member of the rotator cuff group
coracobrachialis	coracoid process of the scapula	medial side of the humerus at mid-shaft	flexes and adducts the arm	musculocutaneous nerve (C5,6)	the musculocutaneous nerve passes through the coracobrachialis muscle to reach the other arm flexor mm.(biceps brachii and brachialis)

17 Deltoid proximal attachments

Deltoid **CLASP**s

Clavicle
Acromion
Spine of scapula`

18Rotator cuff muscles

"The **SITS** muscles":
Clockwise from top:
Supraspinatus
Infraspinatus
Teres **minor**
Subscapularis

 19Bicipital groove: attachments of muscles

"The **lady** between **two majors**":
Teres **major** attaches to medial lip of groove.
Pectoralis **major** to lateral lip of groove.
Latissimus (Lady) is on floor of groove, between the 2 majors.

 20Arm fractures: nerves affected by humerus fracture location

ARM fracture:
From superior to inferior:
Axillary: head of humerus
Radial: mid shaft
Median: supracondylar

21 Anatomical spaces of the arm

Quadrangular space

Space bounded by the teres minor m. superiorly, the teres major m. inferiorly, the long head of the triceps brachii m. medially and the humerus laterally.

Axillary n. and the posterior circumflex humeral a. pass through this space.

Scapula

Teres minor

Teres major

Triceps – long head

Humerus

Triangular space

Space bounded by the teres minor m. superiorly, the teres major m. inferiorly and the long head of the triceps brachii m. laterally.

Circumflex scapular vessels are located in this space as they pass from the axilla to the dorsum of the scapula.

Triangular interval

Interval between the teres major m. superiorly, long head of the triceps brachii m. medially and humerus laterally.

Radial n. passes through this interval to get from the axilla to the posterior surface of the humerus.

22 Anterior (flexor) compartment of the arm

Muscles:

Compartment bounded at its posterior extent by the medial and lateral intermuscular septa and the humerus; it is bounded anteriorly, laterally and medially by the brachial fascia.

Forearm flexors - Anterior	**biceps brachii**	short head: tip of the coracoid process of the scapula; long head: supraglenoid tubercle of the scapula	tuberosity of the radius	flexes the forearm, flexes arm (long head), supinates	musculocutaneous nerve (C5,6)	a powerful supinator only if the elbow is flexed
	brachialis	anterior surface of the lower one-half of the humerus and the associated intermuscular septa	coronoid process of the ulna	flexes the forearm		a powerful flexor
	brachioradialis	upper two-thirds of the lateral supracondylar ridge of the humerus	lateral side of the base of the styloid process of the radius	flexes the elbow, assists in pronation & supination	radial nerve	Although brachioradialis is innervated by the nerve for extensors (radial), its primary action is elbow flexion.
Pronators	**pronator quadratus**	medial side of the anterior surface of the distal one-fourth of the ulna	anterior surface of the distal one-fourth of the radius	pronates the forearm	median nerve	pronator quadratus is the deepest muscle in the distal forearm; it works with pronator teres and has the same nerve supply
	pronator teres	common flexor tendon and (deep or ulnar head) from medial side of coronoid process of the ulna	midpoint of the lateral side of the shaft of the radius			median nerve passes between the two heads of origin of pronator teres

23Elbow: muscles that flex it

Three **B**'s **B**end the el**B**ow:
Brachialis
Biceps
Brachioradialis

 24Musculocutaneous nerve: muscles supplied

BBC:
Biceps brachii
Brachialis
Coracobrachialis

 25 Brachioradialis: function, innervation, one relation, one attachment

BrachioRadialis:

- *Function:* It's the Birell[1] Raising muscle, flexes elbow, strongest when wrist is oriented like holding a Birell.
- *Innervation:* Breaks Rule: it's a flexor muscle, But Radial. (Radial nerve usually is for extensors).
- *Important relation:* Behind it is the Radial nerve in the cubital fossa.
- *Attachment:* Attaches to Bottom of Radius.

---

[1] The original was Beer, but I changed it to its non-alcoholic version: Birell (malt beverage – 0% alcohol – horrible taste)

26 Biceps Brachii Muscle Origins

"It's a **short** distance to the **cor**ner. It's a **long** distance to
the **supra**(high)way."
Short head origin on **cor**acoid process
Long head origin on **supra**glenoid cavity.

27 Posterior (extensor) compartment of the arm

Muscles

Compartment bounded at its anterior extent by the
medial and lateral intermuscular septa and humerus; it is
bounded posteriorly, laterally and medially by the
brachial fascia.

Forearm extensors - Posterior	**triceps brachii**	long head: infraglenoid tubercle of the scapula; lateral head: posterolateral humerus & lateral intermuscular septum; medial head: posteromedial surface of the inferior 1/2 of the humerus	olecranon process of the ulna	extends the forearm; the long head extends and adducts arm	**radial nerve**	long head of the triceps separates the triangular and quadrangular spaces (teres major, teres minor and the humerus are the other boundaries); all three heads of origin insert by a common tendon
	anconeus	lateral epicondyle of the humerus	lateral side of the olecranon and the upper one-fourth of the ulna	extends the forearm		none
Supinator	**supinator**	lateral epicondyle of the humerus, supinator crest & fossa of the ulna, radial collateral ligament, annular ligament	lateral side of proximal one-third of the radius	supinates the forearm		deep radial nerve passes through the supinator to reach the posterior compartment of the forearm

28Supination vs. pronation

"**SOUP**-ination": Supination is to turn your arm palm up, as if you are holding a bowl of **soup**.
"**POUR**-nation": Pronation is to turn your arm with the palm down, as if you are **pour**ing out whatever is your bowl.

 29Supination vs. pronation: which is more powerful

Screws were designed to be tightened well by majority of people.
"Righty tighty": to tighten screws you turn to the right. Majority of people are right-handed. Turning right-hand to the right is supination.

30Changes that occur at the level of insertion of the coracobrachialis

- Median n. crosses brachial artery.
- Ulnar n. pierces medial intramuscular septum.
- Radial n. pierces lateral intramuscular septum.
- Medial cutaneous nerves of arm and forearm pierce deep fascia.
- Basilic vein pierces deep fascia.
- Nutrient artery enter the humerus.
- Deltoid tuberosity ends.

31 Brachial artery

Origin – Axillary artery
(At the lower border of teres major)

Profunda brachii: largest branch, follow <u>radial nerve</u> to the posterior compartment.
(Near the origin)

Superior ulnar collateral: follow <u>ulnar nerve</u> to the back of the elbow.
(At the middle)

Nutrient artery:
(level of insertion of coracobrachialis)

Muscular supply:
to anterior Ms. Group.

Inferior ulnar collateral: Enter the posterior compartment then divides into ant. & post. Branches ant. To medial epicondyle
(Near the end)

Termination: *Radial & ulnar arteries in the cubital fossa.*
(Level of the neck of radius)

32 **Brachial artery: recurrent and collateral branches anastomosis**
"**I A**m **P**retty **S**mart"
Inferior ulnar collateral artery goes with **A**nterior ulnar recurrent artery.
Posterior ulnar recurrent artery goes with **S**uperior ulnar collateral artery.
NB: collateral ulnar arise from brachial artery while recurrent ulnar arise from ulnar artery.

 33 **Cubital fossa contents**
MBBR:
From medial to lateral:
Median nerve
Brachial artery
Biceps tendon
Radial nerve

 34 **Elbow: which side has common flexor origin?**
FM (as in FM Radio):
Flexor **M**edial, so Common Flexor Origin is on the medial side.

Forearm

35 **Anterior forearm muscles: superficial group**

There are five, like five digits of your hand.
Place your thumb into your palm, then lay that hand palm
down on your other arm, as shown in diagram. Your 4
fingers now how distribution: spells **PFPF** [pass/fail,
pass/fail]:

- **P**ronator teres
- **F**lexor carpi radialis
- **P**almaris longus
- **F**lexor carpi ulnaris

Your thumb below your 4 fingers shows the muscle which
is deep to the other four: *Flexor digitorum superficialis.*

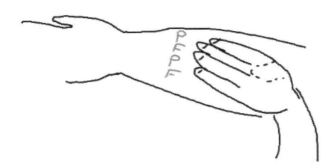

36 Anterior forearm muscles: superficial group

Superficial anterior compartment of forearm	**flexor carpi ulnaris**	common flexor tendon & (ulnar head) from medial border of olecranon & upper 2/3 of the posterior border of the ulna	pisiform, hook of hamate, and base of 5th metacarpal	flexes the wrist, abducts the hand	**ulnar nerve** — the ulnar nerve passes between the two heads of origin of the flexor carpi ulnaris m.
	flexor carpi radialis	common flexor tendon from the medial epicondyle of the humerus	base of the second and third metacarpals		works with the extensor carpi radialis longus and brevis mm. to abduct hand
	flexor digitorum superficialis	humeroulnar head: common flexor tendon; radial head: middle 1/3 of radius	shafts of the middle phalanges of digits 2-5	flexes the metacarpophalangeal and proximal interphalangeal joints	**median nerve** — median nerve travels distally in the forearm on the deep surface of the flexor digitorum superficialis m.
	palmaris longus	common flexor tendon, from the medial epicondyle of the humerus	palmar aponeurosis	flexes the wrist	palmaris longus is absent in about 13% of forearms; it may be present on one side only
	pronator teres	common flexor tendon and (deep or ulnar head) from medial side of coronoid process of the ulna	midpoint of the lateral side of the shaft of the radius	pronates the forearm	median nerve passes between the two heads of origin of pronator teres

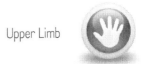

37 Anterior forearm muscles: deep group

Deep anterior compartment of forearm						
	flexor digitorum profundus	posterior border of the ulna, proximal two-thirds of medial border of ulna, interosseous membrane	base of the distal phalanx of digits 2-5	flexes the metacarpophalangeal, proximal interphalangeal and distal interphalangeal joints	median nerve (radial one-half); ulnar nerve (ulnar one-half)	ulnar nerve innervates the portion of profundus that acts on digits 4 & 5 (the ulnar 2 digits)
	flexor pollicis longus	anterior surface of radius and interosseous membrane	base of the distal phalanx of the thumb	flexes the metacarpophalangeal and interphalangeal joints of the thumb	median nerve	the tendon of flexor pollicis longus passes through the carpal tunnel with the other long digital flexor tendons and the median nerve
	pronator quadratus	medial side of the anterior surface of the distal one-fourth of the ulna	anterior surface of the distal one-fourth of the radius	pronates the forearm		pronator quadratus is the deepest muscle in the distal forearm; it works with pronator teres and has the same nerve supply

38 Flexor digitorum muscles: how they insert onto fingers ·

A little rhyme: SS>PPP
Superficialis **S**plits in two,
To **P**ermit **P**rofundus **P**assing through.

39 Posterior forearm muscles: superficial group

Superficial posterior compartment of forearm	extensor carpi ulnaris	common extensor tendon & the middle one-half of the posterior border of the ulna	medial side of the base of the 5th metacarpal	extends the wrist; adducts the hand		works with the flexor carpi ulnaris in adduction of the hand
	extensor digiti minimi	common extensor tendon (lateral epicondyle of the humerus)	joins the extensor digitorum tendon to the 5th digit and inserts into the extensor expansion	extends the metacarpophalangeal, proximal interphalangeal and distal interphalangeal joints of the 5th digit	deep radial nerve	extensor digiti minimi appears to be the ulnar-most portion of extensor digitorum
	extensor digitorum	common extensor tendon (lateral epicondyle of the humerus)	extensor expansion of digits 2-5	extends the metacarpophalangeal, proximal interphalangeal and distal interphalangeal joints of the 2nd-5th digits; extends wrist		the extensor expansion inserts via a central band on the base of the middle phalanx, while lateral & medial slips insert on the distal phalanx
	extensor carpi radialis longus	lower one-third of the lateral supracondylar ridge of the humerus	dorsum of the second metacarpal bone (base)	extends the wrist; abducts the hand	radial nerve	works with the extensor carpi radialis brevis and flexor carpi radialis in abduction of the hand
	extensor carpi radialis brevis	lateral supracondylar ridge of the humerus (common extensor tendon	dorsum of the third metacarpal bone (base)			works with the extensor carpi radialis longus and flexor carpi radialis in abduction of the hand

40 Posterior forearm muscles: deep group

Deep posterior compartment of forearm	**extensor indicis**	interosseous membrane and the posterolateral surface of the distal ulna	its tendon joins the tendon of the extensor digitorum to the second digit; both tendons insert into the extensor expansion	extends the index finger at the metacarpophalangeal, proximal interphalangeal and distal interphalangeal joints		extensor indicis is a deep forearm extensor, whereas extensor digiti minimi is in the superficial layer of extensors
	extensor pollicis brevis	interosseous membrane and the posterior surface of the distal radius	base of the proximal phalanx of the thumb	extends the thumb at the metacarpophalangeal joint	**deep radial nerve**	the tendons of extensor pollicis brevis and abductor pollicis longus make the lateral border of the anatomical snuffbox, in which the radial arterial pulse can be felt
	extensor pollicis longus	interosseous membrane and middle part of the posterolateral surface of the ulna	base of the distal phalanx of the thumb	extends the thumb at the interphalangeal joint		the tendon of extensor pollicis longus hooks around the dorsal radial tubercle; it forms the medial border of the anatomical snuffbox, in which the radial arterial pulse can be felt
	abductor pollicis longus	middle one-third of the posterior surface of the radius, interosseous membrane, mid-portion of posterolateral ulna	radial side of the base of the first metacarpal	abducts the thumb at carpometacarpal joint		the tendons of abductor pollicis longus and extensor pollicis brevis make the lateral border of the anatomical snuffbox

41 Radial nerve: muscles innervated

"**T**ry **A** **B**ig **C**hocolate **C**hip **S**undae, **D**ouble **D**ip **C**herries **A**nd **P**eanuts **P**referably **I**ncluded":

In order of their innervation, proximal to distal:

Triceps
Anconeus
Brachioradialis
ext. **C**arpi radialis longus
ext. **C**arpi radialis brevis
Supinator
ext. **D**igitorum
ext. **D**igiti minimi
ext. **C**arpi ulnaris
Abductor poll. longus
ext. **P**oll. brevis
ext. **P** poll. longus
ext. **I**ndicis

*NB. For the neighboring words that start with the same letter (e.g.: chocolate and chip), notice that the **longer** word in the mnemonic, corresponds to the longer of the two muscle names (ex: ext. carpi radialis **longus** and ext. carpi radialis brevis)*

42 Radial nerve: muscles supplied (simplified)

"**BEST** muscles":
Brachioradialis
Extensors
Supinator
Triceps

43 Ulnar nerve to ulnar artery and radial nerve to radial artery relations

Think "peripheral nerves":
The ulnar nerve is "ulnar" to the ulnar artery.
Radial nerve is "radial" to the radial artery.

Hand

44Carpal bones:

"Sally Lazem Tel3ab Bowling, Teksab Tekhsar Kolo Hals" OR "**S**imply **L**earn **T**he **P**arts **T**hat **T**he **C**arpus **H**as"

Proximal row lateral to medial:
Scaphoid
Lunate
Triquetrium
Pisiform
Distal row, lateral to medial:
Trapezium
Trapezoid
Capate
Hamate

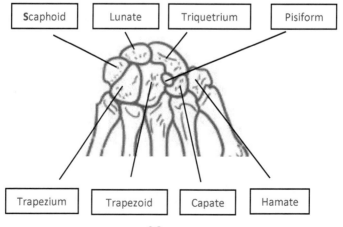

45 Carpal tunnel syndrome causes

MEDIAN TRAP:
Myxedema
Edema premenstrually
Diabetes
Idiopathic
Acromegaly
Neoplasm
Trauma
Rheumatoid arthritis
Amyloidosis
Pregnancy
Mnemonic fits nicely since median nerve is trapped.

46 Intrinsic muscles of hand (palmar surface)

"**A**ll **F**or **O**ne **A**nd **O**ne **F**or **A**ll":
· *Thenar:*
Abductor pollicis longus
Flexor pollicis brevis
Opponens pollicis
Adductor pollicis.
· *Hypothenar:*
Opponens digiti minimi
Flexor digiti minimi
Abductor digiti minimi

47 Thenar muscles

<table>
<tr><td rowspan="2">Thenar muscles</td><td>adductor pollicis</td><td>oblique head: capitate and base of the 2nd and 3rd metacarpals; transverse head: shaft of the 3rd metacarpal</td><td>base of the proximal phalanx of the thumb</td><td>adducts the thumb</td><td>ulnar nerve, deep branch</td><td>deep palmar arch and deep ulnar nerve pass between the two heads of adductor pollicis, which is in the adductor-interosseous compartment</td></tr>
<tr><td>flexor pollicis brevis</td><td>flexor retinaculum, trapezium</td><td>proximal phalanx of the 1st digit</td><td>flexes the carpometacarpal and metacarpophalangeal joints of the thumb</td><td>recurrent branch of the median nerve</td><td>flexor pollicis brevis, abductor pollicis brevis, and opponens pollicis are the three muscles of the thenar compartment of the hand</td></tr>
</table>

48 Hypothenar muscles

<table>
<tr><td rowspan="3">Hypothenar muscles</td><td>flexor digiti minimi brevis</td><td>hook of hamate & the flexor retinaculum</td><td>proximal phalanx of the 5th digit</td><td>flexes the carpometacarpal and metacarpophalangeal joints of the 5th digit</td><td rowspan="3">ulnar nerve, deep branch</td><td>flexor digiti minimi brevis, abductor digiti minimi, and opponens digiti minimi are in the hypothenar compartment of the hand</td></tr>
<tr><td>abductor digiti minimi</td><td>pisiform</td><td>base of the proximal phalanx of the 5th digit on its ulnar side</td><td>abducts the 5th digit</td><td>abductor digiti minimi, flexor digiti minimi brevis, and opponens digiti minimi are located in the hypothenar compartment of the hand</td></tr>
<tr><td>opponens digiti minimi</td><td>hook of hamate and flexor retinaculum</td><td>shaft of 5th metacarpal</td><td>opposes the 5th digit</td><td>opposition is a rotational movement of the 5th metacarpal around the long axis of its shaft</td></tr>
</table>

49 Intermediate muscles

Intermediate muscles	**lumbrical**	flexor digitorum profundus tendons of digits 2-5	extensor expansion on the radial side of the proximal phalanx of digits 2-5	flex the metacarpophalangeal joints, extend the proximal and distal interphalangeal joints of digits 2-5	median nerve (radial 2) via palmar digital nerves & ulnar nerve (ulnar 2) via deep branch	lumbricals, (lumbricus is Latin for "worm") arise from the profundus tendons and have the same pattern of innervation as does the profundus muscle (ulnar and median nn. split the task equally)
	interosseous, dorsal	four muscles, each arising from two adjacent metacarpal shafts	base of the proximal phalanx and the extensor expansion on lateral side of the 2nd digit, lateral & medial sides of the 3rd digit, and medial side of the 4th digit	flex the metacarpophalangeal joint, extend the proximal and distal interphalangeal joints of digits 2-4, abduct digits 2-4 (abduction of digits in the hand is defined as movement away from the midline of the 3rd digit)	ulnar nerve, deep branch	bipennate muscles; remember DAB & PAD - Dorsal interosseous mm. ABduct and Palmar interosseous mm. ADduct - then you can figure out where they must insert to cause these actions
	interosseous, palmar	three muscles, arising from the palmar surface of the shafts of metacarpals 2, 4, & 5	base of the proximal phalanx and extensor expansion of the medial side of digit 2, and lateral side of digits 4 & 5	flexes the metacarpophalangeal, extends proximal and distal interphalangeal joints and adducts digits 2, 4, & 5 (adduction of the digits of the hand is in reference to the midline of the 3rd digit)		unipennate muscles; remember PAD & DAB

39

50 Median and ulnar nerves: common features

- Each supply 1/2 of flexor digitorum profundus.
- Each supplies 2 lumbricals.
- Each has a palmar cutaneous nerve that pops off prematurely.
- Each supplies an eminence group of muscles [ulnar: hypothenar. median: thenar].
- Each enters forearm through two heads [ulnar: heads of flexor carpi ulnaris. - median: heads of pronator teres].
- Each has no branches in upper arm.
- Each makes two fingers claw when cut at wrist.
- Each supplies a palmaris [median: palmaris longus. ulnar: palmaris brevis].

51 Palmaris longus: location, relative to wrist

nerves "The **Palmaris** between **two Palmars**":
Palmaris longus is between the **Palmar** cutaneous branch of Ulnar nerve and **Palmar** cutaneous branch of Median nerve.

52 Median nerve: hand muscles innervated

"The **LOAF** muscles":
Lumbricals 1 and 2
Opponens pollicis
Abductor pollicis brevis
Flexor pollicis brevis

53 Hand: nerve lesions

DR CUMA:
Drop=**R**adial nerve
Claw=**U**lnar nerve
Median nerve=**A**pe hand

This page is left blank intentionally

Chapter 2: Lower Limb

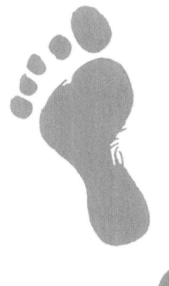

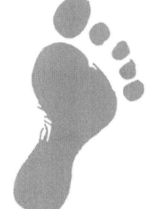

Contents
- Hip
- Thigh
- Knee
- Leg
- Foot

Hip

 1 Hip joint:

Acetabulum articulates with femoral head forming a synovial joint; reinforced by capsular ligaments (iliofemoral, pubofemoral, ischiofemoral and zona orbicularis) and containing acetabular labrum & ligamentum capitis femoris.

 2 Hip posterior dislocation:

Most likely arrangement for one
"Hitting the brake pedal before the accident": You are sitting, so hip is **flexed**, and **adducted** and **medially rotated** so can move your foot away from the gas pedal over to the brake pedal.
Note: car accidents are most likely cause of posterior dislocation because in this position

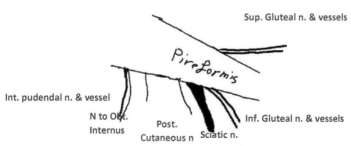 **3** structures passing through greater sciatic foramen

Sup. Gluteal n. & vessels

Int. pudendal n. & vessel

N to Obt. Internus

Post. Cutaneous n

Sciatic n.

Inf. Gluteal n. & vessels

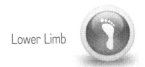

 4Lumbar plexus

Ventral primary rami of spinal nerves L1-L4.

Motor to: muscles of the lower abdominal wall; cremaster m., psoas major and minor m., quadratus lumborum m., iliacus m.; muscles of the anterior and medial thigh and hip.

Sensory to: skin of the lower abdominal wall, skin of the anterior scrotum/labium majus, skin of the anterior and medial thigh and lateral hip.

 5Lumbar plexus – Root values & branches

"2 from 1, 2 from 2, 2 from 3":
2 nerves from **1** root: Ilioinguinal (L1), Iliohypogastric (L1).
2 nerves from **2** roots: Genitofemoral (L1,L2), Lateral Femoral (L2,L3).
2 nerves from **3** roots: Obturator (L2,L3,L4), Femoral (L2,L3,L4).

 6Sacral plexus

Lumbosacral trunk (ventral primary rami of spinal nerves L4-L5), ventral primary rami of spinal nerves S1-S4.

Motor to: muscles of the pelvic diaphragm; muscles of the urogenital diaphragm; muscles of the posterior hip, posterior thigh, leg and foot.

Sensory to: skin of the perineum, posterior thigh, leg and foot (excluding the medial side of the leg and foot).

7 Sacral plexus branches

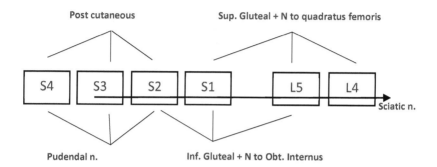

8 Deep tendon reflexes: root supply

"**1,2,3,4,5,6,7,8**":

S**1-2**: ankle
L**3-4**: knee
C**5-6**: biceps, supinator
C**7-8**: triceps

Or (nursery rhyme)
"One, two-- buckle my shoe. Three, four-- kick the door. Five, six-- pick up sticks. Seven, eight-- shut the gate"
S1,2 = ankle jerk L3,4 = knee jerk C5,6 = biceps and brachioradialis C7,8 = triceps

9 Femoral hernia: epidemiology

FEMoral hernias are more common in **FEM**ales.

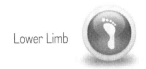

 10 Iliopsoas muscles

	Muscle	Origin	Insertion	Action	Nerve	Notes
Iliopsoas	iliacus	iliac fossa and iliac crest; ala of sacrum	lesser trochanter of femur via iliopsoas tendon	flexes the thigh; if the thigh is fixed it flexes the pelvis on the thigh	femoral nerve	inserts in company with the psoas major m. via the iliopsoas tendon
	psoas major	bodies and transverse processes of lumbar vertebrae		flexes the thigh; flexes & laterally bends the lumbar vertebral column	branches of the ventral primary rami of spinal nerves L2-L4	the genitofemoral nerve pierces the anterior surface of the psoas major m.
	psoas minor	bodies of the T12 & L1 vertebrae	iliopubic eminence at the line of junction of the ilium and the superior pubic ramus	flexes & laterally bends the lumbar vertebral column	branches of the ventral primary rams of spinal nerves L1-L2	absent in 40% of cases

 11 Hip: lateral rotators

"**P-GO-GO-Q**". *From top to bottom:*

Piriformis

       Gemellus superior

       Obturator internus

       Gemellus inferior

       Obturator externus   **Q**uadratus femoris

12hip joint lateral rotators muscles

Lateral Rotators						
	quadratus femoris	lateral border of the ischial tuberosity	quadrate line of the femur below the intertrochanteric crest		nerve to the quadratus femoris m.	the nerve to the quadratus femoris m. also innervates the inferior gemellus m.
	obturator externus	the external surface of the obturator membrane and the superior and inferior pubic rami	trochanteric fossa of the femur	laterally rotates the thigh	obturator nerve	the tendon of the obturator externus m. passes inferior to the neck of the femur to reach its insertion site
	Gemellus inferior	ischial tuberosity	obturator internus tendon		nerve to the quadratus femoris m.	gemellus is a Latin word that means "little twin"
	Gemellus superior	ischial spine			nerve to the obturator internus m.	
	piriformis	anterior surface of sacrum	upper border of greater trochanter of femur	laterally rotates and abducts thigh	ventral rami of S1-S2	piriformis leaves the pelvis by passing through the greater sciatic foramen
	obturator internus	the internal surface of obturator membrane and margin of obturator foramen	greater trochanter on its medial surface above the trochanteric fossa	laterally rotates and abducts the thigh	nerve to the obturator internus m.	The obturator internus m. leaves the pelvis by passing through the lesser sciatic foramen.

13 Hip joint adductors muscles

Observe Three Ducks Pecking Grass

Observe = Obturator
Three Ducks = three Adductors
Pecking = Pectineus
Grass = Gracilis

14 hip joint adductors muscles

Adductors						
	adductor longus	medial portion of the superior pubic ramus	linea aspera of the femur	adducts, flexes, and medially rotates the femur	anterior division of the obturator nerve	the most anterior of the adductor group of muscles
	adductor magnus	ischiopubic ramus and ischial tuberosity	linea aspera of the femur; the ischiocondylar part inserts on the adductor tubercle of the femur	adducts, flexes, and medially rotates the femur; extends the femur (ischiocondylar part)	posterior division of the obturator nerve; tibial nerve (ischiocondylar part)	the ischiocondylar part of adductor magnus is a hamstring muscle by embryonic origin and action, so it is innervated by the tibial nerve
	adductor minimus	lower portion of the inferior pubic ramus	gluteal ridge and upper part of the linea aspera of the femur	adducts and laterally rotates the femur	posterior division of the obturator nerve	adductor minimus m. is the uppermost fibers of the adductor magnus m.
	pectineus	pecten of the pubis	pectineal line of the femur	adducts, flexes, and medially rotates the thigh	femoral nerve and possibly anterior division of the obturator nerve	pectineus often has a dual innervation

gracilis	pubic symphysis and the inferior pubic ramus	medial surface of the tibia (via pes anserinus)	adducts the thigh, flexes and medially rotates the thigh, flexes the leg	anterior division of the obturator nerve	the pes anserinus is the common insertion of the gracilis, sartorius, and semitendinosus mm. (SGT)

15 Gluteus muscles

Gluteus group	gluteus maximus	posterior gluteal line, posterior surface of sacrum and coccyx, sacrotuberous ligament	upper fibers: iliotibial tract; lowermost fibers: gluteal tuberosity of the femur	extends the thigh; laterally rotates the femur	inferior gluteal nerve	gluteus maximus is a site of intramuscular injection
	gluteus medius	external surface of the ilium between posterior and anterior gluteal lines	greater trochanter of the femur	abducts the femur; medially rotates the thigh	superior gluteal nerve	the angle at which the tendons approaches the greater trochanter is anterior to the axis of rotation of the thigh, resulting in medial rotation
	gluteus minimus	External surface of ilium between ant. & inf. gluteal lines				
	tensor fasciae latae	anterior part of the iliac crest, anterior superior iliac spine	iliotibial tract	flexes, abducts, and medially rotates the thigh	superior gluteal nerve	tensor fascia latae redirects the rotational forces of the gluteus maximus m.

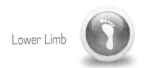

16 collateral circulation around hip joint

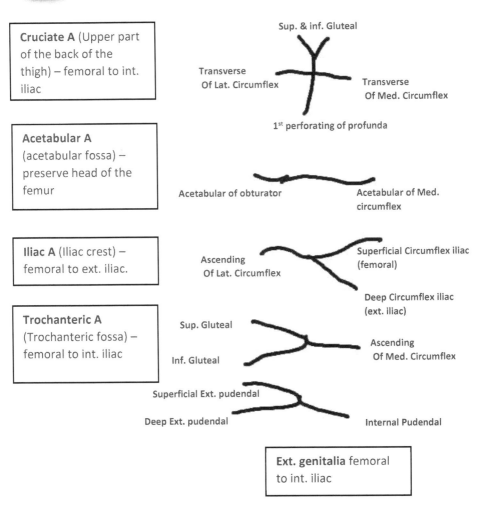

> **Cruciate A** (Upper part of the back of the thigh) – femoral to int. iliac

Sup. & inf. Gluteal

Transverse Of Lat. Circumflex

Transverse Of Med. Circumflex

1st perforating of profunda

> **Acetabular A** (acetabular fossa) – preserve head of the femur

Acetabular of obturator

Acetabular of Med. circumflex

> **Iliac A** (Iliac crest) – femoral to ext. iliac.

Ascending Of Lat. Circumflex

Superficial Circumflex iliac (femoral)

Deep Circumflex iliac (ext. iliac)

> **Trochanteric A** (Trochanteric fossa) – femoral to int. iliac

Sup. Gluteal

Inf. Gluteal

Ascending Of Med. Circumflex

Superficial Ext. pudendal

Deep Ext. pudendal

Internal Pudendal

> **Ext. genitalia** femoral to int. iliac

Thigh

 17 Femoral triangle: boundaries

A musculo-fascial triangle on the anterior surface of the thigh

Femoral triangle is shaped like a "**SAIL**":
Sartorius
Adductor longus
Inguinal **L**igament

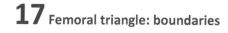 **18** Femoral triangle: contents

NAVY: In order from lateral to medial:
Nerve
Artery
Vein
Y of the groin (the medial side)

 19 Femoral triangle: floor

PIMP
Pectineus
Iliacus
Psoas **M**ajor

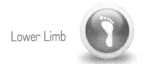

20 Femoral artery

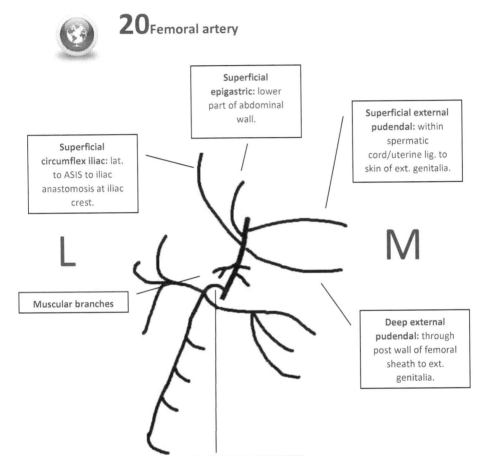

Superficial epigastric: lower part of abdominal wall.

Superficial external pudendal: within spermatic cord/uterine lig. to skin of ext. genitalia.

Superficial circumflex iliac: lat. to ASIS to iliac anastomosis at iliac crest.

L

M

Muscular branches

Deep external pudendal: through post wall of femoral sheath to ext. genitalia.

Profunda Femoris: main supply of the thigh, arise at the post lat aspect 1.5 inch below ing. Lig.

21 Profunda femoris artery

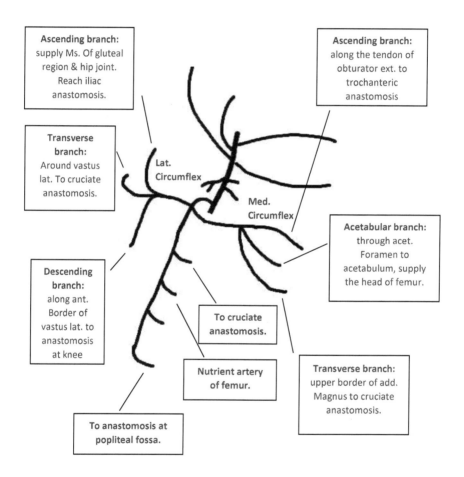

Ascending branch: supply Ms. Of gluteal region & hip joint. Reach iliac anastomosis.

Ascending branch: along the tendon of obturator ext. to trochanteric anastomosis

Transverse branch: Around vastus lat. To cruciate anastomosis.

Lat. Circumflex

Med. Circumflex

Acetabular branch: through acet. Foramen to acetabulum, supply the head of femur.

Descending branch: along ant. Border of vastus lat. to anastomosis at knee

To cruciate anastomosis.

Nutrient artery of femur.

Transverse branch: upper border of add. Magnus to cruciate anastomosis.

To anastomosis at popliteal fossa.

22 Thigh: innervation by compartment

So all muscles in that compartment get innervated by that nerve.

"MAP OF Sciatic":
Medial compartment: **O**bturator
Anterior compartment: **F**emoral
Posterior compartment: **Sciatic**

23 Posterior compartment muscles

A connective tissue compartment that contains the muscles that flex the knee joint and extend the hip joint; its boundaries are: *anterior* - lateral intermuscular septum, femur and fascia between the medial and posterior compartments; *lateral, medial and posterior* - fascia lata.

Posterior comp. (Hamstring Ms.)	**biceps femoris**	long head: ischial tuberosity; short head: lateral lip of the linea aspera	head of fibula and lateral condyle of the tibia	extends the thigh, flexes the leg	long head: tibial nerve; short head: common fibular (peroneal) nerve	one of the "hamstring" muscles
	semimembranosus	upper, outer surface of the ischial tuberosity	medial condyle of the tibia			one of the "hamstring" muscles
	semitendinosus	Lower, medial surface of ischial tuberosity (common tendon with biceps femoris m.)	medial surface of tibia (via pes anserinus)	extends the thigh, flexes the leg	tibial nerve	pes anserinus is the common insertion for the gracilis, sartorius, and semitendinosus mm.

55

24 Anterior compartment muscles

A connective tissue compartment that contains muscles that extend the knee; its boundaries are: *anterior and lateral* - fascia lata of the thigh; *posterior*; femur, medial intermuscular septum and *lateral* intermuscular septum.

<table>
<tr><td rowspan="6" style="writing-mode: vertical">Anterior Comp.</td><td>rectus femoris</td><td>straight head: anterior inferior iliac spine; reflected head: above the superior rim of the acetabulum</td><td>patella and tibial tuberosity (via the patellar ligament)</td><td>extends the leg, flexes the thigh</td><td rowspan="4">femoral nerve</td><td rowspan="4">part of the quadriceps femoris muscle</td></tr>
<tr><td>vastus intermedius</td><td>anterior and lateral surface of the femur</td><td>patella</td><td></td></tr>
<tr><td>vastus lateralis</td><td>lateral intermuscular septum, lateral lip of the linea aspera and the gluteal tuberosity</td><td rowspan="2">patella and medial patellar retinaculum</td><td rowspan="2">extends the leg</td></tr>
<tr><td>vastus medialis</td><td>medial intermuscular septum, medial lip of the linea aspera</td></tr>
<tr><td>sartorius</td><td>anterior superior iliac spine</td><td>medial surface of the tibia (pes anserinus)</td><td>flexes, abducts and laterally rotates the thigh; flexes leg</td><td>sartorius means "tailor"; its actions put the lower limb in the traditional cross-legged seated position of a tailor</td></tr>
</table>

25 Subsartorial canal

A musculo-fascial canal that contains the large neurovascular bundle of the anterior thigh.

Its boundaries are: *anterior* - sartorius m.; *lateral* - vastus medialis m.; *posterior* - adductor longus m. and adductor magnus m.; it *begins* proximally at the inferior angle of the femoral triangle and *ends* distally at the adductor hiatus.

Subsartorial canal contains the femoral a. and v., the saphenous n. and the nerve to the vastus medialis m.; also known as: adductor canal, Hunter's canal.

26 Fascia lata

Deep fascia forming a tubular investment of the thigh.

Fascia lata is thickened laterally to form the iliotibial tract/band; it is connected to the femur by the lateral and medial intermuscular septa which divide the thigh into compartments; Scarpa's fascia attaches to the external surface of the fascia lata inferior to the inguinal ligament.

27 Saphenous hiatus

An opening in the fascia lata located inferior to the inguinal ligament and lateral to the pubic tubercle.

Saphenous hiatus is the site of passage of the greater saphenous vein which joins the femoral vein; it is closed by the cribriform fascia.

Knee

28 knee joint

Synovial joint formed as follows: femoral condyles articulate with tibial condyles; reinforced by intracapsular ligaments (anterior cruciate & posterior cruciate), a capsular ligament (tibial collateral ligament), and an extracapsular ligament (fibular collateral ligament); contains medial & lateral menisci.

29 Popliteal fossa: muscles arrangement

The two Semi's go together, Semimembranosus and Semitendinosus.

The **Membranous** is **Medial** and since the two semis go together, Semitendinosus is also medial.

Therefore, Biceps Femoris has to be lateral.

Of the semi's, to remember which one is superficial: the **Tendinosus** is on **Top**.

30 Popliteal fossa:

Medial to lateral arrangement
"**S**erve **A**nd **V**olley **N**ext **B**all":

Semimembranosus/ **S**emitendinosus
Artery
Vein
Nerve
Biceps femoris
Lateral and medial heads of Gastrocnemius are inferior borders.

31 Cruciate ligaments: insertions

PAMS APPLES:
Posterior [passes] Anterior [inserts] Medially.
Anterior [passes] Posteriorly [inserts] Laterally.

32 M. & L. Meniscus

Medial meniscus intra-articular disc within knee joint between medial femoral condyle & medial tibial condyle; attached to tibial collateral ligament, coronary ligament, & intercondylar eminence.
Lateral meniscus intra-articular disc within knee joint between lateral femoral condyle & lateral tibial condyle; attached to coronary ligament & intercondylar eminence

33 Genu valgum vs. genu vargum

Genu val**GUM** (knock-knee): knees are **GUM**med together.
Varum (bowleg) is the other by default, or **Far** rhymes with **Var**, so knees are **far** apart.

34 Ossification ages

"**E**very **P**otential **A**natomist **S**hould **K**now **W**hen"
When they ossify, in order of increasing year:
Elbow: **16** years
Pelvis, **A**nkle: **17** years
Shoulder, **K**nee: **18** years
Wrist: **19** years

Leg

35 Tibia vs. fibula:

Which is lateral?
The FibuLA is LAteral.

36 Anterior compartment

A connective tissue compartment that contains muscles that dorsiflex the ankle; its boundaries are: tibia, fibula, interosseous membrane, anterior intermuscular septum.
Anterior compartment of the leg contains the tibialis anterior m., extensor hallucis longus m., extensor digitorum longus m., fibularis tertius m.; it also contains the anterior tibial a. and the deep fibular n.; also known as: extensor compartment of the leg.

37 Leg: anterior muscles of leg

"**T**he **H**ospitals –**A**re **N**ot **D**irty **P**laces" or "Tom, Harry AND Peter"
T: **T**ibialis anterior
H: extensor **H**allucis longus
A: anterior tibial **A**rtery
N: deep fibular **N**erve
D: extensor **D**igitorum longus
P: **P**eroneus tertius [fibularis tertius]

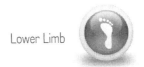

38Leg: anterior muscles

Anterior comp. (Leg)	**tibialis anterior**	lateral tibial condyle and the upper lateral surface of the tibia	medial surface of the medial cuneiform and the 1st metatarsal	dorsiflexes and inverts the foot	acts as both an antagonist (dorsiflexion/plantar flexion) and a synergist (inversion) of the tibialis posterior m.
	fibularis (peroneus) tertius	distal part of the anterior surface of the fibula	dorsum of the shaft of the 5th metatarsal bone	everts the foot	fibularis tertius is in the anterior compartment of the leg, not the lateral compartment (which contains fibularis longus and brevis)
	extensor digitorum longus	lateral condyle of tibia, anterior surface of fibula, lateral portion of the interosseous membrane	dorsum of the lateral 4 toes via extensor expansions (central slip inserts on base of middle phalanx, lateral slips on base of distal phalanx)	extends the metatarsophalangeal, proximal interphalangeal and distal interphalangeal joints of the lateral 4 toes	deep fibular (peroneal) nerve
	extensor hallucis longus	middle half of the anterior surface of the fibula and the interosseous membrane	base of the distal phalanx of the great toe	extends the metatarsophalangeal interphalangeal joints of the great toe	One of the muscles involved in anterior compartment syndrome.

39 Lateral compartment

A connective tissue compartment that contains the muscles that evert the ankle joint; its boundaries are: *anterior, lateral and medial* - crural fascia; *posterior* - anterior and posterior intermuscular septa, fibula.

Lateral compartment of the leg contains: fibularis longus m., fibularis brevis m.; superficial fibular n.; also known as: evertor compartment of the leg.

40 Leg: Lateral muscles

Lateral comp. (Leg) – peroneal						
	fibularis (peroneus)	lower one third of the lateral surface of the fibula	tuberosity of the base of the 5th metatarsal	extends (plantar flexes) and everts the foot	superficial fibular (peroneal) nerve	stress fracture of the base of the 5th metatarsal bone is a common runner's injury
	fibularis (peroneus) longus	upper two/thirds of the lateral surface of the fibula	after crossing the plantar surface of the foot deep to the intrinsic muscles, it inserts on the medial cuneiform and the base of the 1st metatarsal bone			fibularis longus lies superficial to the fibularis brevis m. in the lateral compartment of the leg

41 Lower limb peripheral nerve injuries

"**Drop** into a **DEeP PIT** and **shuffle** your way out":
Foot **Drop** results from **D**orsiflexors and **E**vertors paralysis, due to common **P**eroneal nerve lesion.
Plantar flexion and **I**nversion impairment due to **T**ibial nerve lesion, results in a **shuffling** gait.

42 Posterior compartment

A connective tissue compartment that contains the muscles that plantar flex the ankle joint; its boundaries are: *anterior* - tibia, fibula and interosseous membrane; *lateral, medial and posterior* - crural fascia posterior compartment of the leg.

Contains: *superficially* - gastrocnemius m., soleus m., plantaris m.; *deeply* - popliteus m., tibialis posterior m., flexor digitorum longus m., flexor hallucis longus m.; it also contains the posterior tibial a. and v. and the tibial n.

43 Medial malleolus:

Order of tendons, artery, nerve behind it
"**T**om, **D**ick, **A**nd **N**ervous **H**arry":

From anterior to posterior:
Tibialis
Digitorum
Artery
Nerve
Hallucis

Full names for these are: Tibialis Posterior, Flexor Digitorum Longus, Posterior Tibial Artery, Posterior Tibial Nerve, Flexor Hallucis Longus.

Alternatively: "**T**om, **D**ick **AN**d **H**arry".
Alternatively: "**T**om, **D**ick **A**nd **N**ot **H**arry".

44 Leg: Posterior muscles

Posterior comp. (leg) - Superficial	**Gastrocnemius**	femur; medial head: above the medial femoral condyle; lateral head: above the lateral femoral condyle	dorsum of the calcaneus via the calcaneal (Achilles') tendon	flexes leg; plantar flexes foot	the calcaneal tendon of the gastrocnemius and soleus is the thickest and strongest tendon in the body
	soleus	posterior surface of head and upper shaft of the fibula, soleal line of the tibia	dorsum of the calcaneus via the calcaneal (Achilles') tendon	plantar flexes the foot	soleus, gastrocnemius, and plantaris mm. are sometimes called the triceps surae muscle
	plantaris	above the lateral femoral condyle (above the lateral head of gastrocnemius)	dorsum of the calcaneus medial to the calcaneal tendon	flexes the leg; plantar flexes the foot	**tibial nerve** plantaris has a long slender tendon that is equivalent to the tendon of the palmaris longus m. of the arm; its tendon is often called the "freshman nerve" because it is often misidentified by the freshman medical student
	tibialis posterior	interosseous membrane, posteromedial surface of the fibula, posterolateral surface of the tibia	tuberosity of the navicular and medial cuneiform, metatarsals 2-4	plantar flexes the foot; inverts the foot	acts as both an antagonist (dorsiflexion/plantar flexion) and a synergist (inversion) of the tibialis anterior m.

Posterior comp. (Leg) -Deep	popliteus	lateral condyle of the femur	posterior surface of the tibia above soleal line	flexes and rotates the leg medially (with the foot planted, it rotates the thigh laterally)	tibial nerve	has a round tendon of origin; popliteus unlocks the knee joint to initiate flexion of the leg
	flexor digitorum longus	middle half of the posterior surface of the tibia	bases of the distal phalanges of digits 2-5	flexes the metatarsophalangeal, proximal interphalangeal and distal interphalangeal joints of digits 2-5; plantar flexes the foot		flexor digitorum longus in the leg is equivalent to the flexor digitorum profundus m. of the arm
	flexor hallucis longus	lower 2/3 of the posterior surface of the fibula	base of the distal phalanx of the great toe	flexes the metatarsophalangeal and proximal interphalangeal joints of the great toe; plantar flexes the foot		flexor hallucis longus is very important in the "push off" part of the normal gait

45 Inversion vs. eversion muscles in leg

Second letter rule for inversion/eversion:

Eversion muscles:

pErineus longus

pErineus brevis

pErineus terius

Inversion muscles:

tIbialis anterior

tIbialis posterior

46 Muscles: potentially absent

Muscles which may be absent but may be important:
6 P's:

Palmaris longus [upper limb]
Plantaris [lower limb]
Peroneus tertius [lower limb]
Pyramidalis [anterior abdominal wall]
Psoas minor [posterior abdominal wall]
Platesma [Neck]

Foot

 47 Tarsal bones of ankle

"**T**iger **C**ubs **N**eed **MILC**":
Superior, then clockwise on right foot:

Talus
Calcaneus
Navicular
Medial cuneiform
Intermediate cuneiform
Lateral cuneiform
Cuboid

 48 Tarsal tunnel: contents

"**T**iny **D**ogs **A**re **N**ot **H**unters":
From superior to inferior:
T: **T**ibialis posterior
F: flexor **D**igitorum longus
A: posterior tibial **A**rtery
N: tibial **N**erve
       H: flexor **H**allucis longus

 49 Interossei muscles: actions of dorsal vs. planter in foot

"**Pad** and **DAb**":
The **Pl**anter **Ad**duct and the **D**orsal **Ab**duct. *Use your **hand** to **dab** with a **pad**.*

50Foot muscles

Dorsal gp. (Foot)	**extensor digitorum brevis**	superolateral surface of the calcaneus	extensor expansion of toes 1-4	extends toes 1-4	deep fibular (peroneal) nerve	the part of the extensor digitorum brevis that goes to the great toe is called the extensor hallucis brevis m.
Planter gp. (Layer 1)	**abductor hallucis**	medial side of the tuberosity of calcaneus	medial side of the base of the proximal phalanx of the great toe (hallux)	abducts the great toe; flexes the metatarsophalageal joint	medial plantar nerve	abductor hallucis forms the medial margin of the sole of the foot
	flexor digitorum brevis	tuberosity of the calcaneus, plantar aponeurosis, intermuscular septae	base of the middle phalanx of digits 2-5 after splitting to allow passage of the flexor digitorum longus tendons	flexes the metatarsophalangeal & proximal interphalangeal joints of digits 2-5		flexor digitorum brevis in the foot is equivalent to the flexor digitorum superficialis m. of the arm
	abductor digiti minimi	medial and lateral sides of the tuberosity of the calcaneus	lateral side of the base of the proximal phalanx of the 5th digit	abducts the 5th toe; flexes the metatarsophalageal joint	lateral plantar nerve	abductor digiti minimi forms the lateral margin of the sole of the foot

Planter gp. (Layer 2)	quadratus plantae	anterior portion of the calcaneus and the long plantar ligament	tendons of the flexor digitorum longus m.	assists the flexor digitorum longus in flexing the toes	lateral plantar nerve	the quadratus plantae m. changes the line of force of the flexor digitorum longus m. to bring it in line with the long axis of the foot
	lumbricals (foot)	tendons of the flexor digitorum longus	medial side of the extensor expansion of digits 2-5	flex the metatarsophalan geal joint, extend the proximal interphalangeal & distal interphalangeal joints of digits 2-5	medial (1st) lumbrical: medial plantar nerve; lateral three lumbricals: lateral plantar nerve	the lumbricals of the foot have the same action on the toes that the lumbricals in the hand have on the fingers
Planter gp. (Layer 3)	flexor hallucis brevis	cuboid, lateral cuneiform, medial side of the first metatarsal	medial belly: medial side of proximal phalanx of the great toe; lateral belly: lateral side of the proximal phalanx of the great toe	flexes the metatarsophalan geal joint of the great toe	medial plantar nerve (lateral belly occasionally receives innervation from the lateral plantar nerve)	each tendon of insertion contains a sesamoid bone
	adductor hallucis	oblique head: bases of metatarsals 2-4; transverse head: heads of metatarsals 3-5	lateral side of base of the proximal phalanx of the great toe	adducts the great toe (moves it toward midline of the foot; i.e. Toward the 2nd digit)	deep branch of the lateral plantar nerve	the plantar arterial arch passes superior to the oblique head of adductor hallucis
	flexor digiti minimi brevis	base of 5th metatarsal bone	lateral side of base of proximal phalanx of 5th digit	flexes the metatarsophalan geal joint of the 5th digit	lateral plantar nerve	

Planter gp. (Layer 4)	dorsal interosseous (foot)	shafts of adjacent metatarsal bones	bases of the proximal phalanges for digit 2 (both sides) & digits 3,4 (lateral side)	abduct digits 2-4 (move these digits away from midline as defined by a plane passing through the 2nd digit); flex the metatarsophalangeal joints and extend the interphalangeal joints of those digits	deep branch of the lateral plantar nerve	four in number; remember DAB (Dorsal interossei ABduct) and PAD (Plantar interossei ADduct), then logic can tell you where these muscles insert
	plantar interosseous	base and medial side of metatarsals 3-5	bases of proximal phalanges and extensor expansions of digits 3-5	adduct digits 3-5 (move these digits toward the midline of the foot as defined by a plane through the second digit); flex the metacarpophalangeal and extend interphalangeal joints of digits 3-5	deep branch of the lateral plantar nerve	remember PAD (Plantar interossei ADduct) and DAB (Dorsal interossei ABduct), and logic will tell you where these muscles must insert

 51 Plantar region of foot

AFA 222 FAF

Layer 1: Abductor Hallucis, Flexor digitorum brevis, Abductor digiti minimi

Layer 2: Two tendons (Flexor Hallucis longus, flexor digitorum longus), two muscles
(Lumbricals, quadratus plantae)

Layer 3: Flexor Hallucis brevis, Adductor Hallucis (oblique and transverse heads), Flexor
digiti minimi brevis

Chapter 3: Thorax

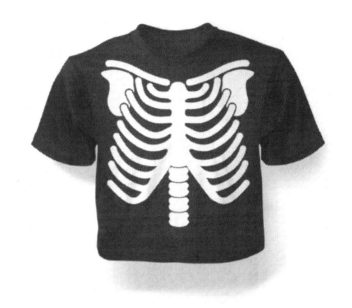

Contents
- Thoracic cage
- Mediastinum
- Viscera

Thoracic cage

1Vertebrae: recognizing a thoracic from lumbar

Examine vertebral body shape:
Thoracic is **heart**-shaped body since your **heart** is in your
thorax.
Lumbar is **kidney-bean** shaped since **kidneys** are in **lumbar** area.

2Thorax: landmarks

Sternal angle: a protrusion on the anterior thoracic wall at the junction of the manubrium and body of the sternum (manubriosternal symphysis). It is the location of the attachment of t the costal cartilage of the 2nd rib to the sternum; an imaginary horizontal plane through the sternal angle passes through the T4/T5 intervertebral disc and marks the inferior boundary of the superior mediastinum.

Suprasternal notch: the notch located at the superior border of the manubrium of the sternum, between the sternal ends of the clavicles, also known as: *jugular notch*.

Thoracic inlet: the opening at the superior end of the rib cage through which cervical structures enter the thorax; bounded by the T1 vertebral body, both of the 1st ribs and their costal cartilages, and the manubrium of the sternum. Thoracic inlet marks the boundary between the neck and the superior mediastinum; also known as: *superior thoracic aperture.*

Thoracic outlet: the opening at the inferior end of the rib cage through which thoracic structures exit the thorax; it is bounded by the T12 vertebral body, both 12th ribs, the costal cartilages of ribs 7-12, and the xiphisternal joint. Thoracic outlet is closed by the respiratory diaphragm which is attached at its boundary; also known as: *inferior thoracic aperture.*

3 Intercostal muscles

Intercostal muscles						
	external intercostal	lower border of a rib within an intercostal space	upper border of the rib below, coursing, downward and forward	keeps the intercostal space from blowing out or sucking in during respiration	intercostal nerves (T1-T11)	11 in number; they extend from the tubercle of the rib to the costochondral junction; continuous with the external intercostal membrane anteriorly
	innermost intercostal	Lower border of rib above	upper borders of rib below	keeps the intercostal space from blowing out or sucking in during respiration		innermost intercostal mm. have the same fiber direction as the internal intercostal mm., the only difference being that they lie deep to the intercostal neurovascular bundle
	internal intercostal	Floor of costal groove of rib above	upper border of rib below, coursing downward and backward	keeps the intercostal space from blowing out or sucking in during respiration		11 in number; they extend from the margin of the sternum to the angle of the rib; continuous posteriorly with the internal intercostal membrane

4Intercostal muscles: extent & fibers direction

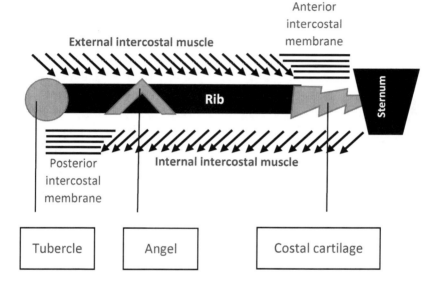

 5Rib costal groove: order of intercostal blood vessels and nerve

VAN:
From superior to inferior:
Vein
Artery
Nerve

6 Intercostal nerves

11 pairs of nerves arise from the ventral primary rami of spinal nerves T1-T11. T12 nerve gives the subcostal nerve. Only 3rd to 6th intercostal nerves are typical nerves with course & branches as follow.

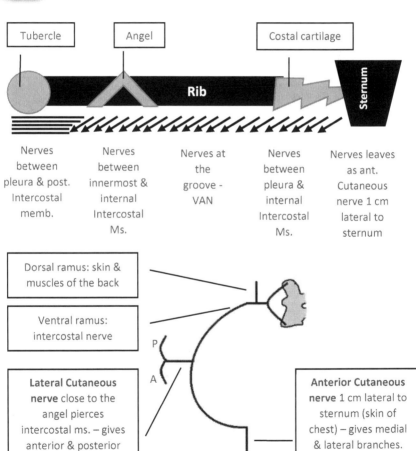

Tubercle	Angel		Costal cartilage	

Rib — Sternum

| Nerves between pleura & post. Intercostal memb. | Nerves between innermost & internal Intercostal Ms. | Nerves at the groove - VAN | Nerves between pleura & internal Intercostal Ms. | Nerves leaves as ant. Cutaneous nerve 1 cm lateral to sternum |

Dorsal ramus: skin & muscles of the back

Ventral ramus: intercostal nerve

Lateral Cutaneous nerve close to the angel pierces intercostal ms. – gives anterior & posterior branches.

Anterior Cutaneous nerve 1 cm lateral to sternum (skin of chest) – gives medial & lateral branches.

75

7 Typical vs. atypical intercostal nerves

	T1	T2	T3 – T6	T7 – T11	T12
Deviation from typical nerves	No cutaneous branches Most of this ramus shares in **brachial plexus**	Its lateral cutaneous branch is called **intercostobrachial** nerve and have no ant. & post. Branches – runs in the **axilla**, supply skin of its floor and upper medial arm	Typical	Leaves intercostal spaces and run forward & downward to supply skin of anterior abdominal wall	Subcostal nerve

8 Thoracic cage: relations to the important venous structures

Behind the **sternoclavicular** joints: the brachiocephalic veins begin.

Behind the **1st costal cartilage** on the right the superior vena cava begins.

Behind the **2nd costal cartilage** on the right the azygos vein ends.

Behind the **3rd costal cartilage** on the right the superior vena cava ends.

9 Internal thoracic (Mammary) artery

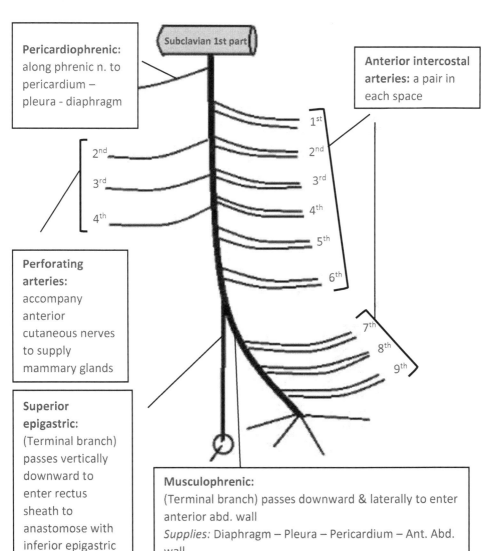

Pericardiophrenic: along phrenic n. to pericardium – pleura - diaphragm

Subclavian 1st part

Anterior intercostal arteries: a pair in each space

1st
2nd
3rd
4th

1st
2nd
3rd
4th
5th
6th
7th
8th
9th

Perforating arteries: accompany anterior cutaneous nerves to supply mammary glands

Superior epigastric: (Terminal branch) passes vertically downward to enter rectus sheath to anastomose with inferior epigastric

Musculophrenic:
(Terminal branch) passes downward & laterally to enter anterior abd. wall
Supplies: Diaphragm – Pleura – Pericardium – Ant. Abd. wall

Mediastinum

10 Posterior mediastinum: Contents

DATES:
Descending aorta
Azygos and hemiazygous veins
Thoracic duct
Esophagus
Sympathetic trunk/ganglia

11 Posterior mediastinum structures

There are 4 birds:
The esopha**GOOSE** (esophagus)
The va**GOOSE** nerve
The azy**GOOSE** vein
The thoracic **DUCK** (duct)

12 Vagus nerve: path into thorax

"I **Left** my **Aunt** in **Vegas**":
Left Vagus nerve goes **Ant**erior descending into the thorax.

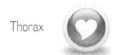

13 Superior mediastinum: contents

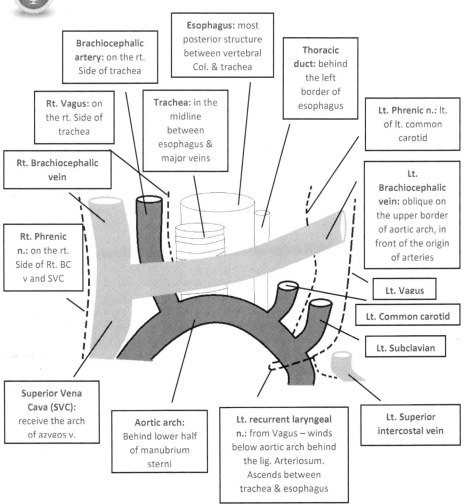

Brachiocephalic artery: on the rt. Side of trachea

Esophagus: most posterior structure between vertebral Col. & trachea

Thoracic duct: behind the left border of esophagus

Rt. Vagus: on the rt. Side of trachea

Trachea: in the midline between esophagus & major veins

Lt. Phrenic n.: lt. of lt. common carotid

Rt. Brachiocephalic vein

Lt. Brachiocephalic vein: oblique on the upper border of aortic arch, in front of the origin of arteries

Rt. Phrenic n.: on the rt. Side of Rt. BC v and SVC

Lt. Vagus

Lt. Common carotid

Lt. Subclavian

Superior Vena Cava (SVC): receive the arch of azygos v.

Aortic arch: Behind lower half of manubrium sterni

Lt. recurrent laryngeal n.: from Vagus – winds below aortic arch behind the lig. Arteriosum. Ascends between trachea & esophagus

Lt. Superior intercostal vein

14 Superior mediastinum: contents

PVT Left BATTLE:
Phrenic nerve
Vagus nerve
Thoracic duct
Left recurrent laryngeal nerve (not the right)
Brachiocephalic veins
Aortic arch (and its 3 branches)
Thymus
Trachea
Lymph nodes
Esophagus

15 Aortic arch: major branch order[1]

"Know your **ABC'S**":
Aortic arch gives rise to:
Brachiocephalic trunk
left **C**ommon **C**arotid
left **S**ubclavian

16 Diaphragm innervation

"**3, 4, 5** keeps the diaphragm alive":
Diaphragm innervation is cervical roots **3**, **4**, and **5**.

---

[1] *NB. Beware though trick question of 'What is first branch of aorta?' Technically, it's the coronary arteries.*

17 Sternal angel

These events happen:

- 2nd costal cartilage attached to the sternum
- Ascending aorta ends
- Aortic arch begins and ends
- Descending aorta begins
- Trachea divides to rt. And lt. bronchi
- Pulmonary trunk divides to rt. And lt. pulmonary arteries
- Azygos vein drains into the superior vena cava
- Thoracic duct crosses to the left border of the esophagus
- Medial borders of both lungs oppose each other in the midline

18 Thoracic duct: relation to azygos vein and esophagus

"The **duck** between **2 gooses**":

Thoracic **duct** (duck) is between 2 gooses, azy**gos** and esopha**gus**.

Viscera

 19Pleura surface markings

"All the even ribs, in order:
2,4,6,8,10,12 show its route":
Rib**2**: sharp angle inferiorly
Rib**4**: the left pleura does a lateral shift to accommodate heart
Rib**6**: both diverge laterally
Rib**8**: midclavicular line
Rib**10**: midaxillary line
Rib**12**: the back

 20Bronchi: which one is more vertical?

"Inhale a **bite**,
goes down the **right**":
Inhaled objects more likely to lodge in right bronchus, since it is the one that is more vertical.

 21Bronchial tree

Primary bronchus: first branch of the air conducting system arising from the bifurcation of the trachea at T4/T5 intervertebral disc. They are paired, right and left; one primary bronchus enters the hilum of each lung; the right primary bronchus is shorter, larger in diameter and

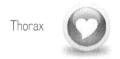

more vertically oriented than the left so that aspirated foreign bodies tend to lodge in the right primary bronchus.

Secondary bronchus: arising from the primary bronchus. There are 3 secondary bronchi in the right lung: upper, middle, lower; there are 2 secondary bronchi in the left lung: upper, lower; also known as: *lobar bronchi.*

Tertiary bronchus: arising from the secondary (lobar) bronchus. there are 10 tertiary bronchi in the right lung: branching from the right superior lobar bronchus - apical, anterior, posterior; branching from the right middle lobar bronchus - medial, lateral; branching from the right inferior lobar bronchus - superior, anterior basal, posterior basal, medial basal, lateral basal; there are 8 tertiary bronchi in the left lung: branching from the left superior lobar bronchus - apicoposterior, anterior; branching from the lingular bronchus (off of the superior lobar bronchus) - superior lingular, inferior lingular; branching from the inferior lobar bronchus - superior, anteromedial basal, posterior basal, lateral basal; also known as: *segmental bronchi.*

22 Atrioventricular valves

"**LAB RAT**":
Left **A**trium: **B**icuspid
Right **A**trium: **T**ricuspid

23 Cross section in the heart

Diaphragmatic surface

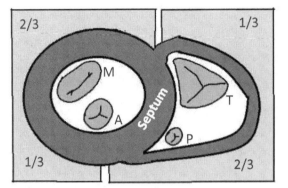

Left

Right

Sternocostal surface

24 Heart – Venous drainage

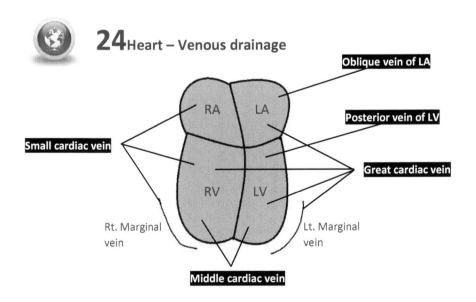

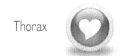

25 Heart – Arterial supply

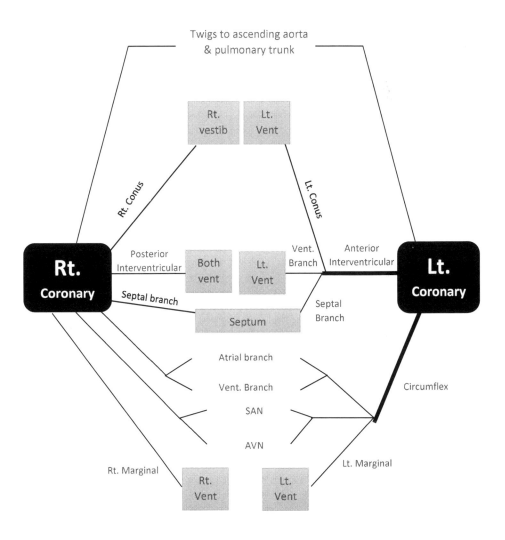

This page was left blank intentionally

Chapter 4: Abdomen & Pelvis

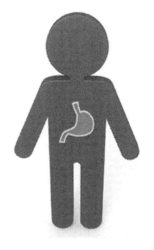

Contents
- Wall
- Vessels
- Viscera

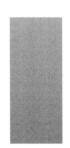

Wall

 1Anterior abdominal wall muscles

Anterior abdominal wall muscles						
	external abdominal oblique	lower 8 ribs	linea alba, pubic crest & tubercle, anterior superior iliac spine & anterior half of iliac crest	flexes and laterally bends the trunk	intercostal nerves 7-11, subcostal, iliohypogastric and ilioinguinal nerves	the inguinal ligament is a specialization of the external abdominal oblique aponeurosis; the external spermatic fascia is the external abdominal oblique muscle's contribution to the coverings of the testis and spermatic cord
	internal abdominal oblique	thoracolumbar fascia, anterior 2/3 of the iliac crest, lateral 2/3 of the inguinal ligament	lower 3 or 4 ribs, linea alba, pubic crest			anterior fibers of internal abdominal oblique course up and medially, perpendicular to the fibers of external abdominal oblique; the cremaster muscle and fascia is the internal abdominal oblique muscle's contribution to the coverings of the testis and spermatic cord
	transversus abdominis	lower 6 ribs, thoracolumbar fascia, anterior 3/4 of the iliac crest, lateral 1/3 of inguinal ligament	linea alba, pubic crest and pecten of the pubis	compresses the abdomen		transversus abdominis muscle does not contribute to the coverings of the spermatic cord and testis; transversalis fascia, the deep fascia that covers the inner surface of the transversus abdominis, forms the internal spermatic fascia
	rectus abdominis	pubis and the pubic symphysis	xiphoid process of the sternum and costal cartilages 5-7	flexes the trunk	intercostal nerves 7-11	rectus sheath contains rectus abdominis and is formed by the aponeurosis of external and internal oblique and transversus abdominis mm.

2 Oblique muscles: direction of externals vs. internals

"Hands in your pockets":
When put hands in your pockets, fingers now lie on top of external oblique and fingers point their direction of fibers: down and towards midline.
Note: "oblique" tells that must be going at an angle.
Internal oblique are at right angles to external.

3 Abdominal muscles

"Spare **TIRE** around their abdomen":

> **T**ransversus abdominis
> **I**nternal abdominal oblique
> **R**ectus abdominis
> **E**xternal abdominal oblique

4 Topographical landmarks

Arcuate line: anatomical feature on the inner surface of the abdominal wall; a fascial line in the transverse plane approximately 1/2 of the distance from the umbilicus to the pubic symphysis.
 Arcuate line is the point at which the posterior lamina of the rectus sheath ends and transversalis fascia lines the inner surface of the rectus abdominis m.

Linea Alba: anatomical feature on the midline of the anterior abdominal wall; an aponeurotic band that extends from the xiphoid process to the pubic symphysis.

Linea Alba is formed by the combined abdominal muscle aponeuroses; it is used for midline abdominal incisions to avoid major nerves or vessels.

 5 Rectus sheath

Above arcuate line

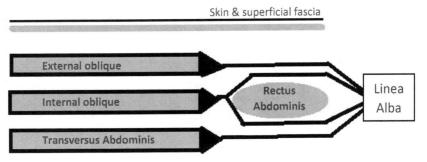

Below arcuate line

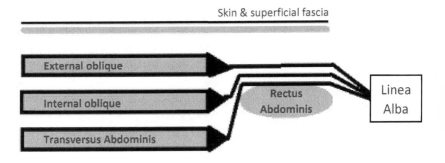

6 Inguinal canal: walls

"MALT: 2M, 2A, 2L, 2T":
Starting from superior, moving around in order to posterior:

Superior wall (roof): 2 **M**uscles:

- Internal oblique **M**uscle
- Transverse abdominis **M**uscle

Anterior wall: 2 **A**poneuroses:

- **A**poneurosis of external oblique
- **A**poneurosis of internal oblique

Lower wall (floor): 2 **L**igaments:

- Inguinal **L**igament
- Lacunar **L**igament

Posterior wall: 2**T**s:

- **T**ransversalis fascia
- Conjoint **T**endon

7 Inguinal canal: walls

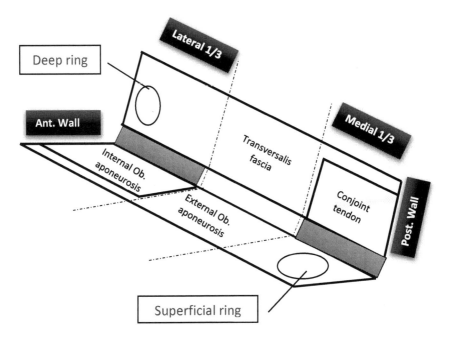

 8 Inguinal canal: roof & floor

Internal oblique muscle – transversus abdominis		
Roof		
Floor		
Inguinal ligament		
Iliopubic track (lat. 1/3)		Lacunar ligament (med 1/3)

9 Spermatic cord contents

"**3** arteries, **3** nerves, **3** other things":

> **3** arteries: testicular, ductus deferens, cremasteric.
> **3** nerves: genital branch of the genitofemoral, cremasteric, autonomics.
> **3** other things: ductus deferens, pampiniform plexus, lymphatics.

10 Spermatic cord contents

"**P**iles **D**on't **C**ontribute **T**o **A** **G**ood **S**ex **L**ife":

> **P**ampiniform plexus
> **D**uctus deferens
> **C**remasteric artery
> **T**esticular artery
> **A**rtery of the ductus deferens
> **G**enital branch of the genitofemoral nerve
> **S**ympathetic nerve fibers
> **L**ymphatic vessels

11 Scrotum layers

"**S**ome **D**ays **E**ddie **C**an **I**rritate **P**eople **V**ery **T**horoughly":

> **S**kin
> **D**artos layer
> **E**xternal spermatic fascia
> **C**remaster muscle
> **I**nternal spermatic fascia
> **P**arietal tunica vaginalis
> **V**isceral tunica vaginalis
> **T**unica albuginea

12 Dartos & Cremaster

Dartos & Cremaster	**cremaster**	inguinal ligament	forms thin network of muscle fascicles around the spermatic cord and testis (or around the distal portion of the round ligament of the uterus)	elevates testis (not well developed in females)	genital branch of the genitofemoral nerve	the cremaster m. is internal abdominal oblique muscle's contribution to the coverings of the spermatic cord and testis; the cremasteric reflex may be elicited by stroking the medial thigh (where the femoral branch of the genitofemoral n. distributes cutaneously)
	dartos	subcutaneous connective tissue of the scrotum and the penis (or labium majus and clitoris)	skin of the scrotum and penis (or labium majus and clitoris)	elevates testis (tenses the skin of the pudendal region in the female)	postganglionic sympathetic nerve fibers arriving via the ilioinguinal nerve and the posterior scrotal nerve	the dartos elevates the testis in response to cold (it is modified arrector pili fibers, or the goose-bump muscles)

13 Sperm pathway through male reproductive tract

SEVEN UP:

Seminiferous tubules
Epididymis
Vas deferens
Ejaculatory duct
Nothing
Urethra
Penis

14 Umbilicus

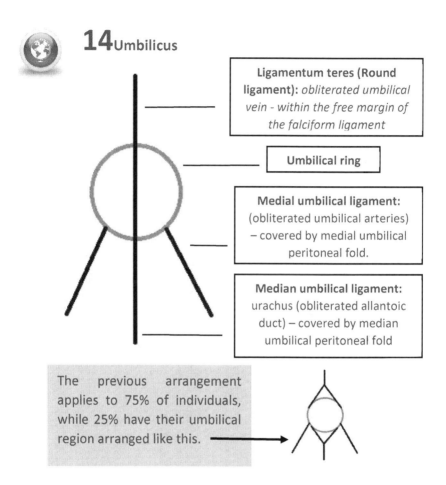

Ligamentum teres (Round ligament): *obliterated umbilical vein - within the free margin of the falciform ligament*

Umbilical ring

Medial umbilical ligament: (obliterated umbilical arteries) – covered by medial umbilical peritoneal fold.

Median umbilical ligament: urachus (obliterated allantoic duct) – covered by median umbilical peritoneal fold

The previous arrangement applies to 75% of individuals, while 25% have their umbilical region arranged like this.

15 Umbilical peritoneal folds

Median: covering Urachus
Medial: covering medial umbilical ligaments

Lateral: covering inferior epigastric vessels

16 L4 landmark

2 items "B4U" [before you]:
Bifurcation of aorta
L4
Umbilicus

17 Three danger areas in the inguinal region[1]

The Triangle of Doom: is formed by the gonadal vessels laterally and the ductus deferens medially. The apex is the deep inguinal ring. Within this triangle are: external iliac vessels, deep circumflex iliac vein, genital branch of the genitofemoral nerve, and the femoral nerve (deep).

The Triangle of Pain: is formed by the iliopubic tract inferolaterally and the gonadal vessels superomedially. It contains a lot of nerves, such as lateral femoral cutaneous, anterior femoral cutaneous, femoral branch of genitofemoral, and femoral nerve.

The Circle of Death: is formed by the common iliac vessels, internal and external iliac vessels, obturator vessels, aberrant obturator vessels, and inferior epigastric vessels.

---

[1] This section is related to the laparoscopic anatomy of the inguinal region. Far advanced for undergrads. From Skandalakis' Surgical Anatomy, Chapter 9. Abdominal Wall and Hernias. The McGraw-Hill Companies (2006)

18Hesselbach's triangle

Site of the direct inguinal hernia.

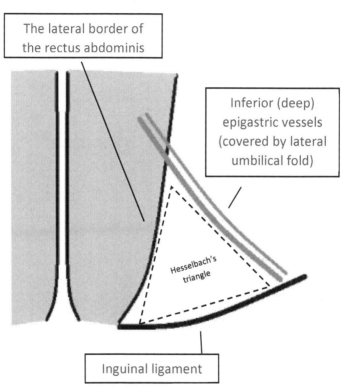

The lateral border of the rectus abdominis

Inferior (deep) epigastric vessels (covered by lateral umbilical fold)

Hesselbach's triangle

Inguinal ligament

Vessels

19 **Descending abdominal aorta: seven divisions**

"**S**ometimes **I**ntestines **G**et **R**eally **S**tretched **C**ausing **L**eakage":

> **S**uprarenal [paired]
> **I**nferior mesenteric
> **G**onadal [paired]
> **R**enal [paired]
> **S**uperior mesenteric
> **C**eliac
> **L**umbar [paired]

20 **Spinal cord: length in vertebral column**

SCULL:
Spinal **C**ord **U**ntil **L2** (**LL**).

21 **Bifurcation vertebral landmarks**

A bifurcation occurs on 4th level of each vertebral column:
C4: bifurcation of common carotid artery
T4: bifurcation of trachea
L4: bifurcation of aorta

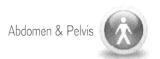

22 Aorta: paired vs. unpaired branches

Aorta Man

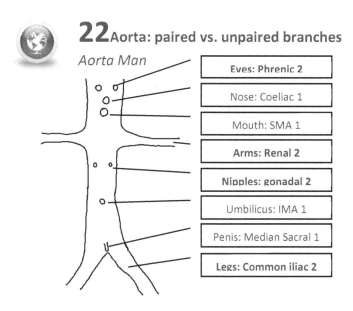

| Eyes: Phrenic 2 |
| Nose: Coeliac 1 |
| Mouth: SMA 1 |
| **Arms: Renal 2** |
| **Nipples: gonadal 2** |
| Umbilicus: IMA 1 |
| Penis: Median Sacral 1 |
| **Legs: Common iliac 2** |

23 Diaphragm apertures: spinal levels

"**C**ome **E**nter the **A**bdomen:
Vena **C**ava [8] **E**sophagus [10] **A**orta [12]

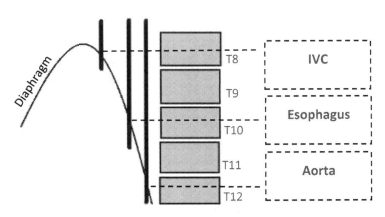

24 Abdominal aorta & IVC[2] - levels

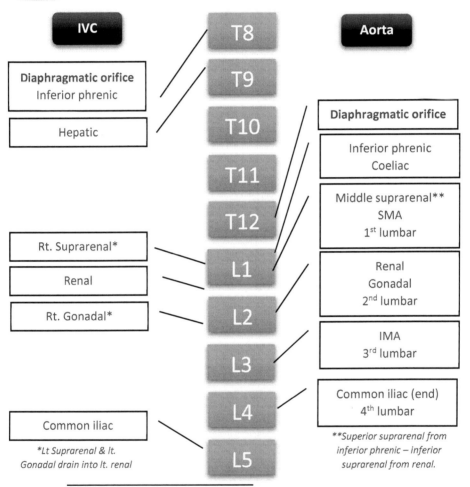

IVC — T8 — **Aorta**

IVC	Level	Aorta
Diaphragmatic orifice Inferior phrenic	T8	
	T9	
Hepatic	T10	**Diaphragmatic orifice**
	T11	Inferior phrenic Coeliac
	T12	Middle suprarenal** SMA 1st lumbar
Rt. Suprarenal*	L1	Renal Gonadal 2nd lumbar
Renal		
Rt. Gonadal*	L2	IMA 3rd lumbar
	L3	
	L4	Common iliac (end) 4th lumbar
Common iliac	L5	

*Lt Suprarenal & lt. Gonadal drain into lt. renal

**Superior suprarenal from inferior phrenic – inferior suprarenal from renal.

[2] IVC doesn't have unpaired branches – the equivalent veins of the unpaired branches of the aorta drains into the portal circulation.

25 Inferior vena cava tributaries

"**I L**ike **T**o **R**ise **S**o **H**igh":
Illiacs
Lumbar
Testicular
Renal
Suprarenal
Hepatic vein.
Think of the IVC wanting to rise high up to the heart.

26 Coeliac trunk: branches

Left **H**and **S**ide (**LHS**):
Left gastric artery
Hepatic artery
Splenic artery

27 Coeliac trunk: detailed branches

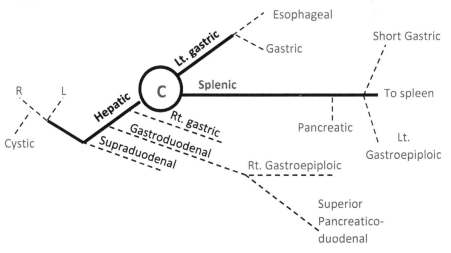

28 Blood supply of the stomach[3]

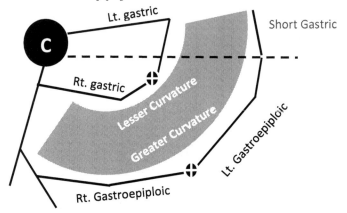

*NB1: **Gastroepiploic vessels** (also named gastro-omental vessels) supply also the greater omentum.*

*NB2: **Short gastric vessels** reach the stomach by passing through the gastrosplenic ligament; they are usually 4-5 in number.*

*NB3: stomach has **a very reach blood supply** due to its rich anastomotic network. This is a double edged weapon during surgery. On the bright side; the stomach can withstand ligation of up to 4 of its 5 named arteries, but on the other hand, ligation of these arteries may fail to stop bleeding from a gastric ulcer[4].*

---

[3] See the previous section (map 27) for details of origin of each artery.
[4] Skandalakis' Surgical Anatomy, Chapter 15. Stomach. The McGraw-Hill Companies (2006).

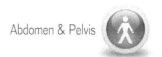

 # 29 Superior mesenteric artery

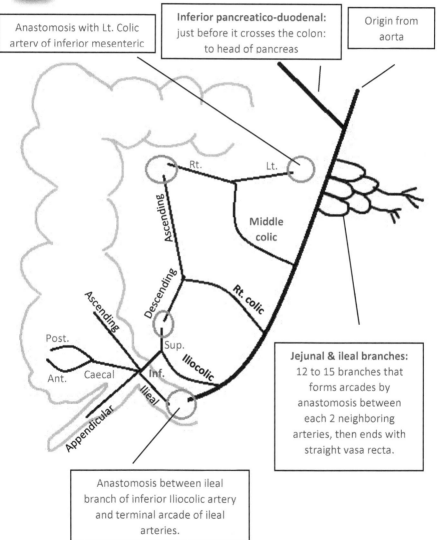

Anastomosis with Lt. Colic artery of inferior mesenteric

Inferior pancreatico-duodenal: just before it crosses the colon: to head of pancreas

Origin from aorta

Rt.

Lt.

Ascending

Middle colic

Descending

Rt. colic

Ascending

Post.

Sup.

Ant.   Caecal   Inf.

Iliocolic

Ileal

Appendicular

Jejunal & ileal branches: 12 to 15 branches that forms arcades by anastomosis between each 2 neighboring arteries, then ends with straight vasa recta.

Anastomosis between ileal branch of inferior Iliocolic artery and terminal arcade of ileal arteries.

30 Inferior mesenteric artery

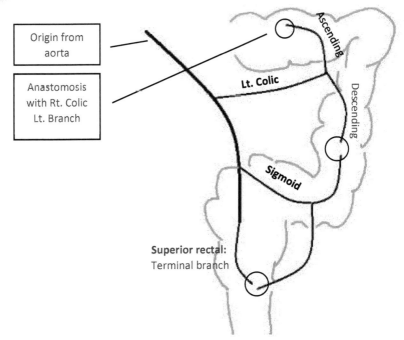

Origin from aorta

Anastomosis with Rt. Colic Lt. Branch

Ascending

Lt. Colic

Descending

Sigmoid

Superior rectal: Terminal branch

31 Ureter to ovarian/testicular artery relation

"**Water under** the bridge":
The **ureters** (which carry water), are **posterior** to the ovarian/testicular artery.
· Clinically important, since a common surgical error is to cut ureter instead of ovarian artery when removing uterus.

32 Branches of Internal Iliac Artery

"I Love Going Places In My Very Own Underwear[5]":

Ileolumbar

Lateral sacral

Gluteal (superior and inferior)

Pudendal (internal)

Inferior vesicle (uterine in females)

Middle rectal

Vaginal

Obturator

Umbilical

33 Internal iliac artery: posterior branch

PILS:

Posterior branch

Iliolumbar

Lateral sacral

Superior gluteal

34 Internal pudendal branches

"I Pee Pee, But Don't Dump!":

Inferior rectal

Posterior scrotal (or labial)

Perineal

Bulb

Deep artery

Dorsal artery

---

[5] But still, under your pants. So, no offence!!

35 Portal vein – The Gazelle[6]

Imagine the portal vein and its branches as a jumping gazelle.

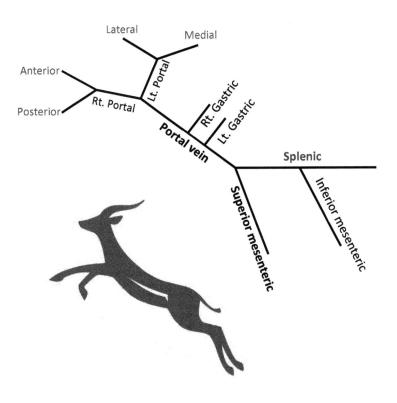

---

[6] The gazelle resemblance of portal branches is originally a radiological example of the intrahepatic portal branches as they appear in CT-Portography. I made some tweaks to include the extrahepatic vessels as well.

Viscera

36 **Retroperitoneal structures list:**

CURSED PAK
(Think of it like back, but distorted by the curse)

Colon (ascending & descending)
Ureters
Rectum
Suprarenal glands
Esophagus (anterior & left covered)
Duodenum (half)

Pancreas
Aorta & IVC
Kidneys

37 **Trans-pyloric plane**

Level of the body of L1

Can be identified by asking the supine patient to sit up without using their arms. The plane is located where the lateral border of the rectus muscle crosses the costal margin.

Structures in the Trans-pyloric plane

- Pylorus stomach – hence the name.
- Left kidney hilum (L1- left one!) The right kidney is shifted 1.5 cm lower than the left by the liver.
- Fundus of the gallbladder.
- Neck of pancreas.
- Superior mesenteric artery (SMA).
- Portal vein (PV).
  Both SMA & PV runs behind the neck of pancreas.
- Left and right colic flexure.
- Root of the transverse mesocolon.
  The transvers colon itself is mobile and hanged lower by its mesocolon – it is fixed by the Lt. and Rt. Colic flexure
- 2nd part of the duodenum.
- Duodenojejunal flexure.
  Both 2nd and 4th part of the duodenum are on the same level creating its G shape.
- Upper part of conus medullaris.
- Spleen.

 38Structures in the Trans-pyloric plane

The pylorus between 2 duodenums (2nd & 4th parts). Behind it the neck of pancreas covering 2 vessels (SMA & PV). In front of it the transverse mesocolon between 2 colonic flexures (Rt. & Lt.).
On the far left 2 organs (spleen and kidney) and on the Right the gall bladder. And related to the L1 vertebra itself: the conus medullaris.

39 Duodenum: lengths of parts

"Counting **1 to 4** but staggered":
1st part: **2** inches
2nd part: **3** inches
3rd part: **4** inches
4th part: **1** inch

40 Lesser sac

Part of the peritoneal cavity located posterior to the stomach and lesser omentum. Also known as *omental bursa.* Opened into the greater sac via the epiploic foramen.

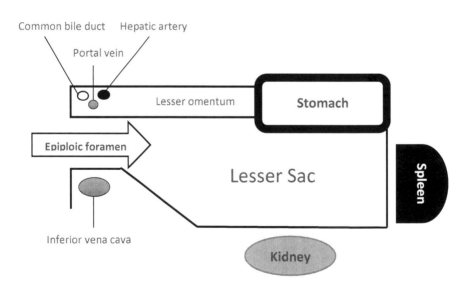

41 Stomach bed

Posterior relations of the stomach

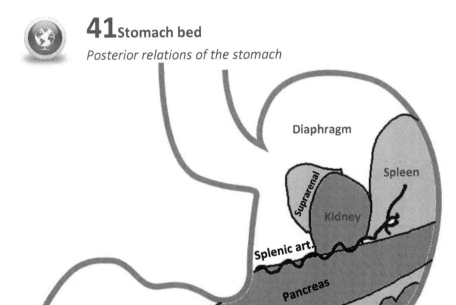

42 Stomach bed structures

Super Kids **Are Sp**ending **M**any **Da**ys **P**laying **C**ards

    Suprarenal gland (Lt.)

    Kidney (Lt.)

    Artery (splenic)

    Spleen

    Mesocolon (Transverse)

    Diaphragm

    Pancreas (Body)

    Colon (Lt. Colic flexure)

43 Stomach anterior relations

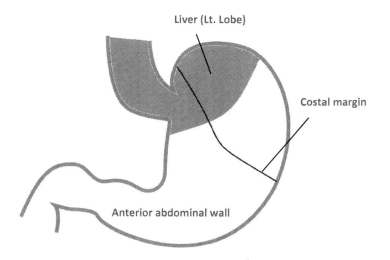

Liver (Lt. Lobe)

Costal margin

Anterior abdominal wall

44 Meckel's diverticulum[7] details

The rule of 2

2 inches long.

2 feet from end of ileum.

2 times more common in men.

2% occurrence in population.

2 types of tissues may be present (intestinal or gastric)

*NB. "**di-**" means "**two**", so **diverticulum** is the thing with all the **two**s.*

---

[7] Congenital anomaly

45 Colon – mobile or fixed

Transverse colon is mobile along the transverse mesocolon

Phrenicocolic ligament between the diaphragm and the splenic flexure. This ligament directs the direction of the enlarging spleen in pathological conditions towards the midline

Caecum is mobile

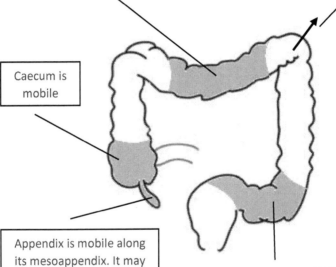

Appendix is mobile along its mesoappendix. It may be located in one of the following positions:

- Pelvic
- Postileal
- Preileal
- Subcecal
- Retrocecal

The mobility of sigmoid can result in the famous condition of *sigmoid volvulus*, if it was twisted on the sigmoid mesocolon

46 Spleen: dimensions, weight, surface anatomy

"**1,3,5,7,9,11**":
Spleen dimensions are **1** inch x **3** inches x **5** inches.
Weight is **7** ounces[8].
It underlies ribs **9** through **11**.

47 Spleen: Ligaments

Phrenicocolic ligament: not attached to the spleen, the lower pole of the spleen is resting on it

Splenophrenic ligament: upper pole of the spleen to the diaphragm

Ligaments on the ventral surface of the spleen:
- **Gastrosplenic**
- **Splenorenal**
- **Pancreaticosplenic**
- **Presplenic fold**

Upper pole

Spleen parietal surface

Lower pole

Splenocolic ligament: lower pole of the spleen to the splenic flexure

---

[8] 1 ounce = 28 grams

48Gastrosplenic & splenorenal ligaments

Cross section

Gastrosplenic ligament: a double layer of peritoneum between the hilum of the spleen and the fundus of the stomach, contains short gastric & Lt. Gastroepiploic vessels.

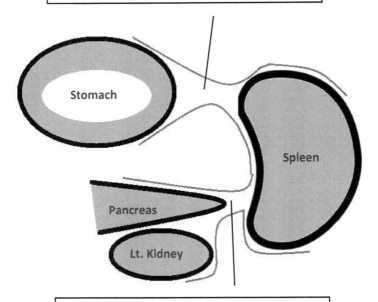

Splenorenal ligament: a double layer of peritoneum between the hilum of the spleen and the fundus of the stomach, contain splenic vessels and the tail of pancreas

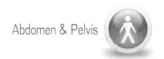

 49 Kidney hilum at trans-pyloric plane [L1]

> **L-1** goes through hilum of only **1** kidney, and it's the **L**eft one.

 50 Kidney anterior relations

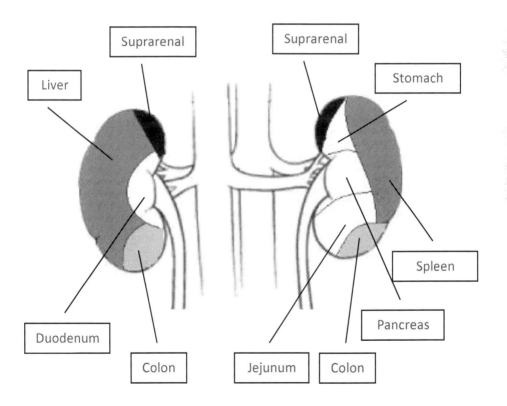

51 Posterior relation of the kidney

LMNOPQRST
L Lateral arcuate ligament
M Medial arcuate ligament
N Nerves
  • Subcostal nerves
  • Iliohypogastric nerve
  • Ilioinguinal nerve
O Oh! Diaphragm!!!
P Psoas major
Q Quadratus lumborum
R Rib

52 Posterior relation of the kidney - numbers

1-2-3-4 All Boys Need Muscle
1 **A**ll = **1 A**rtery
2 **B**oys = **2 B**ones
3 **N**eed = **3 N**erves
4 **M**uscle = **4 M**uscles

53 Liver: side with ligamentum venosum/ caudate lobe vs. side with quadrate lobe/ ligamentum teres

"**VC** goes with **VC**":
The **V**enosum and **C**audate is on same side as **V**ena **C**ava [posterior]. Therefore, quadrate and teres must be on anterior by default.

54 Liver anatomical vs. surgical lobes

Around the year 300 BC Herophilus of Chalcedon[9] wrote the first known anatomic description of liver.

> *"In some [animals] the liver does not have lobes at all but is round and undifferentiated. In some however it has two, in some more, and in many four and in some more lobes."*

Since then the debate went on. Many scientists offered theories on how many lobe the liver has. This debate may be due to the peculiarity of the liver morphology or the complicity of its vascular supply.

Anyway, while anatomists settled for the 4 lobed liver (caudate, quadrate, right and left lobes) based on the external morphology, surgeons prefer the 8 segments system described by Claude Couinaud in 1954.

In this system; the right and left lobe are no longer separated by the falciform ligament, but instead by the Couinaud line; an imaginary line passing through the IVC and the gall bladder. The later system can be denoted sometimes as the vascular liver lobes.

---

[9] Skandalakis' Surgical Anatomy, Chapter 19. Liver. The McGraw-Hill Companies (2006).

55 **Liver inferior markings showing right/left lobe vs. vascular divisions**

There's a **H**epatic "**H**" on inferior of liver. One vertical stick of the H is the dividing line for anatomical right/left lobe and the other vertical stick is the divider for vascular halves.

Stick that divides the liver into vascular halves is the one with vena cava impression (since vena cava carries blood, it's fortunate that it's the divider for blood halves).

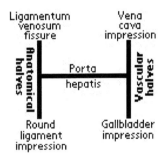

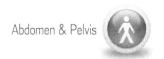
 # 56 Liver – the Couinaud segments[10]

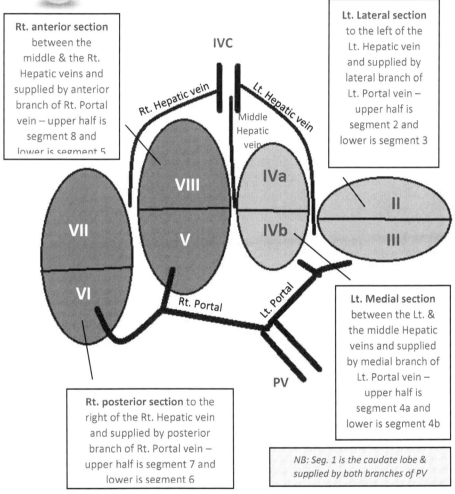

Rt. anterior section between the middle & the Rt. Hepatic veins and supplied by anterior branch of Rt. Portal vein – upper half is segment 8 and lower is segment 5

Lt. Lateral section to the left of the Lt. Hepatic vein and supplied by lateral branch of Lt. Portal vein – upper half is segment 2 and lower is segment 3

IVC

Rt. Hepatic vein

Lt. Hepatic vein

Middle Hepatic vein

VIII

IVa

VII

V

IVb

II

III

VI

Rt. Portal

Lt. Portal

PV

Lt. Medial section between the Lt. & the middle Hepatic veins and supplied by medial branch of Lt. Portal vein – upper half is segment 4a and lower is segment 4b

Rt. posterior section to the right of the Rt. Hepatic vein and supplied by posterior branch of Rt. Portal vein – upper half is segment 7 and lower is segment 6

NB: Seg. 1 is the caudate lobe & supplied by both branches of PV

---

[10] A far advanced piece of information, but as I am a visceral surgeon, I could not resist writing it.

57 Broad ligament: contents

BROAD:

    Bundle (ovarian neurovascular bundle)
    Round ligament
    Ovarian ligament
    Artefacts (vestigial structures)
    Duct (oviduct)

58 Female pelvic organs' blood supply

"**3** organs, **each get 2** blood supplies":

    Uterus: uterine, vaginal.
    Rectum: middle rectal, inferior rectal [inferior
    rectal is the end of pudendal].
    Bladder: superior vesical, inferior vesical.

59 Anal and urethral sphincters

S 2, 3 and 4
Keep the pee off the floor!
You can remember that the second, third and
fourth sacral nerve roots supply these sphincters
from this simple rhyme.

Chapter 5: Head & Neck

Contents
- Cranium
- Face & Jaw
- Neck

Cranium

 1Scalp: layers

SCALP
S skin
C connective tissue
A aponeurosis
L loose connective tissue
P periosteum

 2Scalp: nerve supply

GLASS:
Greater occipital/ **G**reater auricular
Lesser occipital
Auriculotemporal
Supratrochlear
Supraorbital

 3Occipitofrontalis

occipitofrontalis						
	frontalli	aponeurosis	skin of the eyebrows	elevates the eyebrows and	temporal branches of the facial nerve (VII)	the frontalis and occipitalis muscles are two bellies of the occipitofrontalis muscle; also known as: epicranius m.
	occipita	superior nuchal line	aponeurosis	wrinkles the forehead	posterior auricular branch of the facial nerve (VII)	

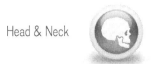

4 Cavernous sinus: relations

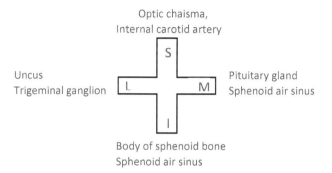

Optic chaisma,
Internal carotid artery

Uncus
Trigeminal ganglion

Pituitary gland
Sphenoid air sinus

Body of sphenoid bone
Sphenoid air sinus

5 Cavernous sinus: communications

Below stated the anterior, posterior, inferior & superior communications. Medially, the 2 cavernous sinuses communicates with each other by 3 intercavernous sinuses.

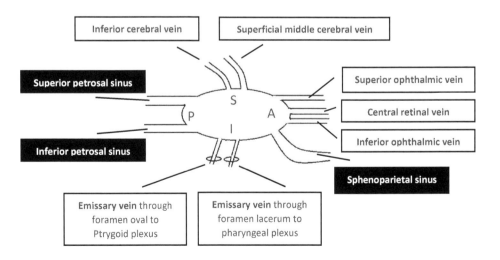

Inferior cerebral vein

Superficial middle cerebral vein

Superior petrosal sinus

Superior ophthalmic vein

Central retinal vein

Inferior petrosal sinus

Inferior ophthalmic vein

Sphenoparietal sinus

Emissary vein through foramen oval to Ptrygoid plexus

Emissary vein through foramen lacerum to pharyngeal plexus

6 Cavernous sinus: contents

O TOM CAT:

O TOM are lateral wall components, in order from superior to inferior.

CA are the components within the sinus, from medial to lateral. CA ends at the level of T from O TOM. *See the diagram.*

> **O**cculomotor nerve (III)
> **T**rochlear nerve (IV)
> **O**phthalmic nerve (V1)
> **M**axillary nerve (V2)
> **C**arotid artery
> **A**bducent nerve (VI)
> **T**: When written, connects to the T of OTOM.

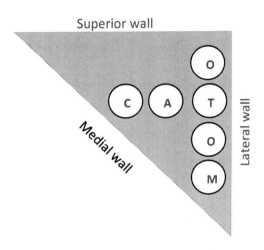

7 **Pituitary gland: relations**

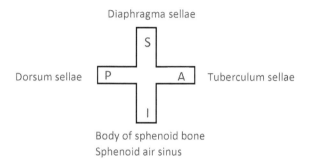

Diaphragma sellae

Dorsum sellae — Tuberculum sellae

Body of sphenoid bone
Sphenoid air sinus

 8 **Orbit: bones of medial wall**

"**M**y **L**ittle **E**ye **S**its in the orbit":
        Maxilla (frontal process)
        Lacrimal
        Ethmoid
        Sphenoid (body)

 9 **Ear: bones of inner ear**

Describes the shape, and relative position (from out to in) of the inner ear bones.

        Take a Hammer: Malleus
        Hit an Indian Elephant: Incus
        It puts its foot in a stirrup: Stapes
        *Alternatively: "**Mail**ing **Inc**ludes **Sta**mps".*

10 Base of the skull foramina

ROS is well known mnemonic for the 3 important foramina of the middle cranial fossa.

Rotundum

Ovale

Spinosum

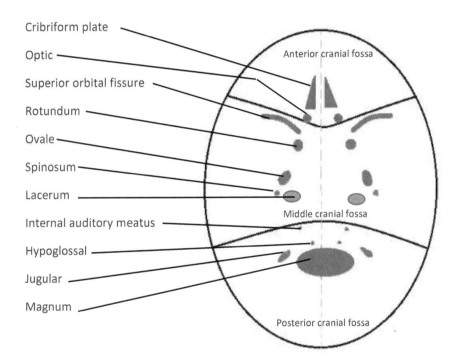

Cribriform plate

Optic

Superior orbital fissure

Rotundum

Ovale

Spinosum

Lacerum

Internal auditory meatus

Hypoglossal

Jugular

Magnum

Anterior cranial fossa

Middle cranial fossa

Posterior cranial fossa

11Foramina: connections & structures passing

Foramen	From	Passing[1]	To
Cribriform plate	Anterior cranial fossa	Olfactory (CN1[2])	Ethmoid air cells – nasal cavity
Optic		Optic (CN2) Ophthalmic artery	Orbit
Superior orbital fissure	Middle cranial fossa	Oculomotor (CN3) Trochlear (CN4) Ophthalmic div. of trigeminal (CN5a) Abducent (CN6)	Orbit (posteromedial)
Rotundum		Maxillary div. of trigeminal (CN5b)	Inferior orbital fissure – pterygopalatine fossa
Ovale		Maxillary div. of trigeminal (CN5b)	The other side of the sphenoid bone medial to tempromandibular joint
Spinosum		Middle meningeal artery Meningeal branch of mandibular nerve	
Lacerum		Part of the course of internal carotid artery	Between body of sphenoid and basal part of occipital bone
Internal auditory meatus	Posterior cranial fossa	Fascial (CN7) Vestibulocochlear (CN8) Labyrinthine artery	Through petrous part of temporal bone, via middle ear to external auditory meatus
Hypoglossal		Hypoglossal (CN12)	Near articular facet of atlanto-occipital
Jugular		Glossopharyngeal (CN9) Vagus (CN10) Accessory (CN11) Sigmoid sinus to Internal jugular vein	Medial to styloid process
Magnum		Medulla oblongata Spinal root of accessory n. Vertebral artery Anterior & posterior spinal arteries	Central vertebral canal

---

[1] Only major structures are mentioned here

[2] CN = cranial nerve

12 Foramen ovale contents

OVALE:

    Otic ganglion (just inferior)

    V3 cranial nerve

    Accessory meningeal artery

    Lesser petrosal nerve

    Emissary veins

 # 13 Foramen ovale contents

Another mnemonic

MALE

    Mandibular nerve

    Accessory meningeal artery

    Lesser petrosal nerve

    Emissary veins

 # 14 Foramen magnum

VAMPIRE

    Vertebral artery

    Anterior spinal artery

    Medulla oblongata

    Posterior Spinal artery

    Its covering (meninges covering of the medulla)

    Root of accessory nerve (spinal root)

    Enough

15 Foramen magnum

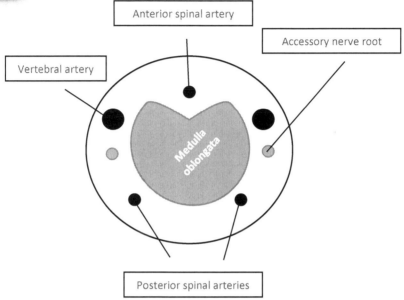

Anterior spinal artery

Accessory nerve root

Vertebral artery

Medulla oblongata

Posterior spinal arteries

16 Foramina of Luschka and Magendie

The roof of the fourth ventricle has three foramina: the medial foramen of Magendie and two foramens of Luschka. They transmit the cerebrospinal fluid into the subarachnoid space.

The locations of these foramina are:

Magendie Medial

Luschka Lateral

17 Jugular foramen

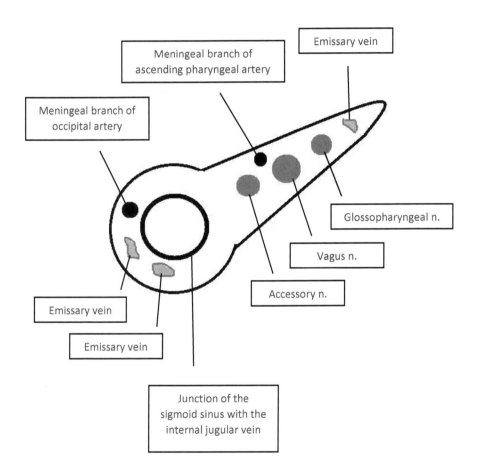

Emissary vein

Meningeal branch of ascending pharyngeal artery

Meningeal branch of occipital artery

Glossopharyngeal n.

Vagus n.

Accessory n.

Emissary vein

Emissary vein

Junction of the sigmoid sinus with the internal jugular vein

18 Superior orbital fissure: structures passing through

"Live Free To See Absolutely No Insult":

- **L**acrimal nerve
- **F**rontal nerve
- **T**rochlear nerve
- **S**uperior branch of Oculomotor nerve
- **A**bducent nerve
- **N**asociliary nerve
- **I**nferior branch of Oculomotor nerve

19 Inferior orbital fissure: Structures passing through

"ZIME"

- **Z**ygomatic nerve
- **I**nfraorbital vessels
- **M**axillary nerve
- **E**missary vein

20 Cranial nerves and eye movements

SALT ME DOWN:

Six Abducts Laterally, Trochlear acts Medially Down. The oculomotor nerve is responsible for everything else.

CN6 = Abducent > supply the lateral rectus only, so abducts the eye.

CN4 = Trochlear > supply the superior oblique only, so it depress the eye (only when the eye is adducted, or moving medially by the medial rectus.

CN3 = oculomotor > supply the other 4 muscles, so responsible for the rest of eye movements.

21Orbit fissures & extraocular muscles

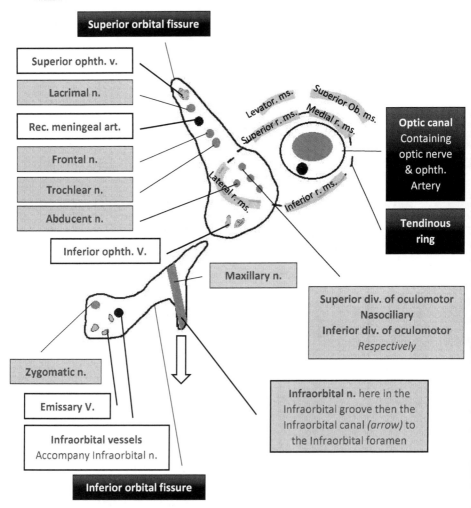

Superior orbital fissure

Superior ophth. v.

Lacrimal n.

Rec. meningeal art.

Frontal n.

Trochlear n.

Abducent n.

Inferior ophth. V.

Levator. ms.

Superior Ob. ms.

Superior r. ms.

Medial r. ms.

Lateral r. ms.

Inferior r. ms.

Optic canal
Containing optic nerve & ophth. Artery

Tendinous ring

Maxillary n.

Superior div. of oculomotor
Nasociliary
Inferior div. of oculomotor
Respectively

Zygomatic n.

Emissary V.

Infraorbital vessels
Accompany Infraorbital n.

Infraorbital n. here in the Infraorbital groove then the Infraorbital canal *(arrow)* to the Infraorbital foramen

Inferior orbital fissure

22 Important foramina content

"Max Returns Mandy's Ovum… May Marry Spinster"

MAX = Maxillary nerve
Returns foramen = Rotundum
  Mandy's = Mandibular nerve
  Ovum = foramen Ovale
May Marry = Middle Meningeal Artery
Spinster = foramen Spinosum

23 Lacrimal nerve course

"Lacrimal's story of 8 L's":
 Lacrimal nerve runs on Lateral wall of orbit above
 Lateral rectus. Then Lets communicating branch join in.
 Then supplies Lacrimal gland. Then Leaves it and
 supplies Lateral upper eye Lid!

24 Brain lobes & its functions

- **Frontal** contains prefrontal (emotions, personality) and precentral (primary and secondary motor) areas.
- **Parietal** contains the primary and secondary somatosensory areas.
- **Temporal** primarily concerned with hearing and memory/learning.
- **Occipital** contains the primary and secondary visual cortex.
- **Limbic** it is the part of the brain responsible for behavior and emotions.

25 Cranial nerves: names & types

Names: Oh, Oh, Oh, To Take A Family Vacation! Go Vegas After Hours.

Sensory or motor: Some say marry money but my brother says big brain matter more.

Nr.	Cranial Nerves	Mnemonic	Type
I	Olfactory	Oh	Some (Sensory)
II	Optic	Oh	Say (Sensory)
III	Oculomotor	Oh	Marry (primarily Motor)
IV	Trochlear	To	Money, (primarily Motor)
V	Trigeminal	Try	But (Both)
VI	Abducent	A	My (primarily Motor)
VII	Facial	Family	Brother (Both)
VIII	Vestibulocochlear	Vacation	Says (Sensory)
IX	Glossopharyngeal	Go	Big (Both)
X	Vagus	Vegas	Brain (Both)
XI	Accessory Nerve	After	Matter (primarily Motor)
XII	Hypoglossal	Hours	More (primarily Motor)

26 Circle of Willis

Meet the weird Mr. Willis!

He has Eyes, hair, face, arms, legs, chest and a penis[3].

Hair = anterior Cerebral	
Eyes = internal carotid	
Face = communicating (Ant. & post)	
Arms = Posterior Cerebral	
Chest as following: Vertebral column: Basilar 1st rib: Superior Cerebellar Ribs: Pontine branches: Last rib: Anterior inferior Cerebellar (AICA)	
Legs = Vertebral	
Penis = Anterior spinal	

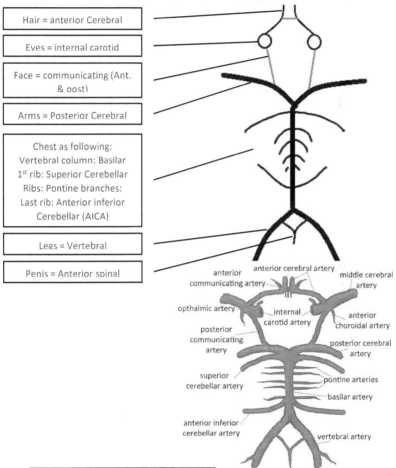

anterior communicating artery — anterior cerebral artery — middle cerebral artery — opthalmic artery — internal carotid artery — anterior choroidal artery — posterior communicating artery — posterior cerebral artery — superior cerebellar artery — pontine arteries — basilar artery — anterior inferior cerebellar artery — vertebral artery

---

[3] Don't you dare mock Mr. Willis unless you found your own Royal College of Surgeons, discover a circle of arteries in the base of the brain and number the cranial nerves as we still do nowadays. **Thomas Willis** (1621 –1675)

Face & jaw

27 Facial nerve: branches after Stylomastoid foramen

"Tow Zombies Borrowed My Car":
Alternatively: "To Zanzibar By Motor Car[4]"

> *From superior to inferior:*
> **T**emporal branch
> **Z**ygomatic branch
> **B**uccal branch
> **M**andibular branch
> **C**ervical branch

28 Bell's palsy: symptoms

BELL's palsy:
> **B**link reflex abnormal
> **E**arache
> **L**acrimation [deficient, excess]
> **L**oss of taste
> **S**udden onset
> **P**alsy of VII nerve muscles
> *NB. All symptoms are unilateral.*

---

[4] Obviously an Indian mnemonic, but it rhymes well, at least to me.

29 Parotid gland – structures exiting its borders

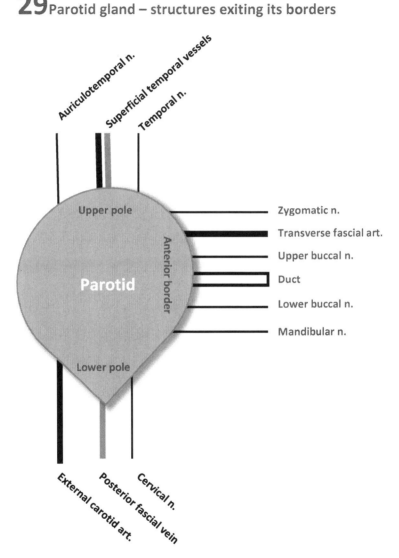

30 Muscles of mastication

Muscles of mastication					
masseter	zygomatic arch and zygomatic bone	lateral surface of the ramus and angle of the mandible	elevates the mandible	A branch named after each muscle from the mandibular division of the trigeminal nerve (V)	a powerful chewing muscle
temporalis	temporal fossa and the temporal fascia	coronoid process of the mandible and the anterior surface of the ramus of the mandible	elevates the mandible; retracts the mandible (posterior fibers)		a powerful chewing muscle; a derivative of the first pharyngeal arch
lateral pterygoid	superior head: greater wing of the sphenoid bone; inferior head: lateral surface of the lateral pterygoid plate	superior head: capsule and & articular disk of the tempromandibular joint; inferior head: neck of the mandible	protracts the mandible; opens the mouth; active in grinding actions of chewing		the only one of the muscles of mastication that opens the mouth; the superior head of lateral pterygoid is sometimes called sphenomeniscus due to its insertion into the disc of the tempromandibular joint
medial pterygoid	medial surface of the lateral pterygoid plate, pyramidal process of the palatine bone, tuberosity of the maxilla	medial surface of the ramus and angle of the mandible	elevates and protracts the mandible		this muscle mirrors the masseter m. in position and action with the ramus of the mandible between the two mm.

 # 31 Pterygoid muscles: function of lateral vs. medial

"Look at how your jaw ends up when saying first syllable of 'Lateral' or 'Medial':

"La": your jaw is now **open**, so Lateral **opens** mouth.

"Me": your jaw is still **closed**, so medial **closes** the mandible.

32 Facial bones

"Virgil Can Not Make My Pet Zebra Laugh!"
Vomer
Conchae
Nasal
Maxilla
Mandible
Palatine
Zygomatic
Lacrimal

33 Mandibular nerve innervated muscles

(Branchial arch 1 derivatives)
"**M.D. My TV**": **M**astication [masseter, temporalis, pterygoids] **D**igastric [anterior belly] **My**lohyoid tensor **T**ympani tensor **V**eli palatini

34 Extrinsic muscles of tongue

(For pro soccer fans)
"**Pa**ris **St**. **Ge**rmain's **Ho**ur":
 Palatoglossus
 Styloglossus
 Genioglossus
 Hyoglossus
NB. PSG is a French soccer team (foreign), hence extrinsic comes to mind.

35 Three important muscles of the face

Muscles of the face						
	buccinator	pterygomandibular raphe, mandible, and the maxilla lateral to the molar teeth	angle of mouth and the lateral portion of the upper and lower lips	pulls the corner of mouth laterally; presses the cheek against the teeth	facial nerve (VII)	although the buccinator is important in mastication, it is innervated by the buccal branch of the facial nerve and NOT by the buccal nerve from V3 (a sensory nerve)
	orbicularis oris	skin and fascia of lips and the area surrounding the lips	skin and fascia of the lips	purses the lips		the "kissing" muscle
	orbicularis oculi	orbital part: medial orbital margin and the medial palpebral ligament; palpebral part: medial palpebral ligament	orbital part: skin of the lateral cheek; palpebral part: lateral palpebral raphe	closes the eyelids		activated involuntarily in the blink reflex; the palpebral part is active in normal blinking and the orbital part is used to forcefully close the eye

Neck

36 Subclavian artery branches

"**V**ery **T**ired **I**ndividuals **S**ip **S**trong **C**offee **S**erved **D**aily":

Vertebral artery
Thyrocervical trunk
---**I**nferior thyroid
---**S**uperficial cervical
---**S**uprascapular
Costocervical
---**S**uperior intercostal
---**D**eep cervical

37 External carotid artery branches

"**S**ome **A**merican **L**adies **F**ind **O**ur **P**yramids **M**ost
Sa**T**isfactory":
Down and upwards

Superior thyroid
Ascending pharyngeal
Lingual
Facial
Occipital
Posterior auricular
Maxillary
Superficial **T**emporal

38 Carotid sheath contents

"**I See 10 CC**'s in the **IV**"

> I See (I.C.) = **I**nternal **C**arotid artery
> 10 = CN **10** (Vagus nerve)
> CC = **C**ommon **C**arotid artery
> IV = **I**nternal Jugular **V**ein

39 Superior thyroid artery branches

"**M**ay **I S**oftly **S**queeze **C**harlie's **G**uitar?"

> **M**uscular
> **I**nfrahyoid
> **S**uperior laryngeal
> **S**ternomastoid
> **C**ricothyroid
> **G**landular

40 External jugular vein: tributaries

PAST:
> **P**osterior external jugular vein
> **A**nterior jugular vein
> **S**uprascapular vein
> **T**ransverse cervical vein

41 Six triangles of the neck – borders & content

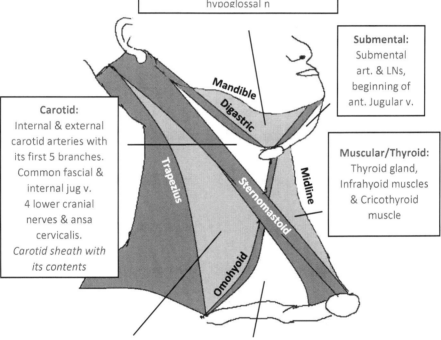

Digastric/submandibular:
submandibular gland, submandibular LN, ant. Fascial vein, fascial art. & hypoglossal n

Submental:
Submental art. & LNs, beginning of ant. Jugular v.

Carotid:
Internal & external carotid arteries with its first 5 branches. Common fascial & internal jug v. 4 lower cranial nerves & ansa cervicalis. *Carotid sheath with its contents*

Muscular/Thyroid:
Thyroid gland, Infrahyoid muscles & Cricothyroid muscle

Occipital:
Accessory nerve, Superficial cervical cutaneous branches of cervical plexus, transverse cervical and suprascapular arteries

Supraclavicular:
Subclavian artery (3rd part), trunks of brachial plexus, & External Jugular Vein

Mandible

Digastric

Trapezius

Sternomastoid

Midline

Omohyoid

42 Cervical plexus: arrangement of the important cutaneous nerves

At the posterior border of the Sternomastoid.
"GLAST":
4 compass points: clockwise from north on the right side of neck:

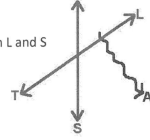

Great auricular
Lesser occipital
Accessory nerve pops out between L and S
Supraclavicular
Transverse cervical

43 Ansa cervicalis nerves

"**GH**ost **TH**ought **S**omeone **ST**upid **SH**ot **I**rene":
Geniohyoid
Thyrohyoid
Superior **O**mohyoid
Sternothyroid
Sternohyoid
Inferior omohyoid

44 Horner's syndrome components

SPAM:
Sunken eyeballs/ **S**ympathetic plexus (cervical) affected
Ptosis
Anhydrosis
Miosis

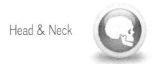

45 Cervical plexus & ansa cervicalis

It is formed of ventral primary rami of spinal nerves C1-C4.

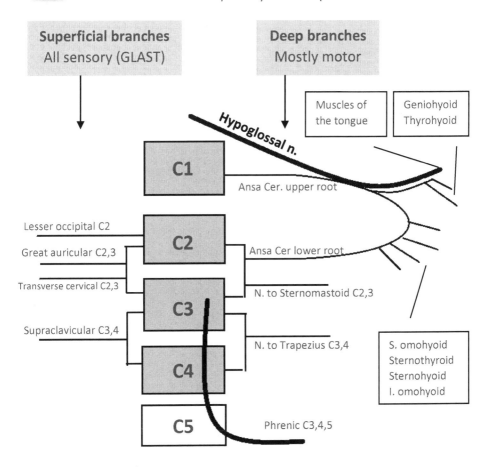

Superficial branches
All sensory (GLAST)

Deep branches
Mostly motor

Muscles of the tongue

Geniohyoid Thyrohyoid

Hypoglossal n.

C1

Ansa Cer. upper root

Lesser occipital C2

C2

Ansa Cer lower root

Great auricular C2,3

Transverse cervical C2,3

N. to Sternomastoid C2,3

C3

Supraclavicular C3,4

N. to Trapezius C3,4

C4

S. omohyoid
Sternothyroid
Sternohyoid
I. omohyoid

C5

Phrenic C3,4,5

NB. Close association of the supraclavicular n. to the phrenic n. results in pain from the respiratory diaphragm referred to the shoulderC2,3 – e.g.in cholecystitis and acute myocardial ischemia pain are referred to rt. & lt. shoulders respectively.

46 Thyroid: isthmus location

It is the constricted midline connection between the lateral lobes of the thyroid gland.

"Rings **2,3,4** - make the **isthmus floor**":
Isthmus overlies tracheal rings **2,3,4**

46 Symptoms of hypothyroidism[5]

Hypothyroidism is 10 times more common in females & occurs mainly in middle life.
Mnemonic: **MOM'S SO TIRED**

> **M**emory loss
> **O**besity
> **M**alar flush/**M**enorrhagia
> **S**lowness
> **S**kin and hair become dry
> **O**nset is gradual
> **T**ired
> **I**ntolerance to cold
> **R**aised blood pressure
> **E**nergy levels are low
> **D**epressed

---

[5] Although those 2 mnemonics (46 &47) are unrelated to anatomy, I chose to include them because both are so helpful. Besides, their topic keeps popping up in every exam through all my study.

47 Symptoms of hyperthyroidism

Mnemonic: **SWEATING**

Sweating
Weight loss
Emotional liability
Appetite is increased
Tremor/**T**achycardia due to AF
Intolerance to heat/**I**rregular menstruation/**I**rritability
Nervousness
Goiter and **G**astrointestinal problems (loose stools/diarrhea)

Made in the USA
Lexington, KY
19 June 2016